ABOUT THE AUTHOR

Dr Lisa Das is a Consultant Gastroenterologist and IBS specialist based in London, with twenty-three years of experience in diagnosing and treating IBS in the US and UK. She currently holds both Board Certification in Gastroenterology (USA) and full accreditation on the UK General Medical Council's Specialist Register in Gastroenterology. As the UK's first Community Gastroenterology Consultant at Bart's Health NHS Trust, where she worked until early 2020, Das has been uniquely well positioned to understand the challenges around IBS encountered by health practitioners and patients alike.

Beyond being outspoken about IBS within the healthcare community, Das has also contributed to TV's *Dr Christian Will See You Now* and has been featured in several *Cosmopolitan* articles shedding light on the disorder. As an expert consultant, Dr Das focuses on providing clinically excellent care with a kind, friendly approach. Her passion for deepening IBS understanding and emphasizing the importance of a strong patient–doctor relationship brings *Managing IBS* to life.

PENGUIN LIFE EXPERTS SERIES

The Penguin Life Experts series equips readers with simple but vital information on common health issues and empowers readers to get to know their own bodies to better improve their health. Books in the series include:

Managing IBS

DR LISA DAS

PENGUIN LIFE

AN IMPRINT OF

PENGUIN BOOKS

PENGUIN LIFE

UK | USA | Canada | Ireland | Australia
India | New Zealand | South Africa

Penguin Life is part of the Penguin Random House group of companies
whose addresses can be found at global.penguinrandomhouse.com.

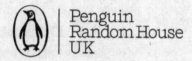

First published 2022
001

Copyright © Dr Lisa Das, 2022

The moral right of the author has been asserted

Set in 12.5/14.75pt Garamond MT Std
Typeset by Jouve (UK), Milton Keynes
Printed and bound in Great Britain by Clays Ltd, Elcograf S.p.A.

The authorized representative in the EEA is Penguin Random House Ireland,
Morrison Chambers, 32 Nassau Street, Dublin D02 YH68

A CIP catalogue record for this book is available from the British Library

ISBN: 978-0-241-53003-0

www.greenpenguin.co.uk

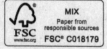

MIX
Paper from
responsible sources
FSC® C018179

Penguin Random House is committed to a
sustainable future for our business, our readers
and our planet. This book is made from Forest
Stewardship Council® certified paper.

To my mum & dad, 'Ami Tomake Bhalobashi.'
You instilled the magical pleasure of active listening,
which I realize now is also an act of love.

And to those who have spoken endlessly to brick walls and
barriers, don't simply be heard – choose to be understood.

Contents

Introduction: What is IBS?

We can all agree that our quality of life is crucial. But when it comes to irritable bowel syndrome (IBS), this can all too often be forgotten.

IBS is a chronic and often debilitating disorder that is known to affect approximately 10 per cent of the global population (although this can vary in different parts of the world). It affects all members of society, regardless of age, sex, race or socioeconomic standing, though women are twice as likely to suffer from IBS worldwide as men, except in India, which surprisingly reports more male prevalence.

Those affected often struggle on with symptoms that can cause pain, discomfort and embarrassment before getting the right help. As a consultant gastroenterologist, I have seen patients try restrictive diets without proper medical guidance, or spend money on expensive tests or supplements to no avail. Others turn to 'Dr Google', with extensive internet searches that can herald confusing and contradictory information. And when they do seek medical help, it can frequently take multiple frustrating appointments with several doctors to get a diagnosis.

Even then, a diagnosis of IBS can in itself be confusing. IBS has no one specific cause: it is what is known as a 'functional problem', so it is not something that shows up through any one test or procedure. The type and severity of symptoms vary from person to person – and even then they may change over time in an individual. There is no single standard treatment. This can be upsetting for some patients, who may believe they aren't being listened to and are instead being given a catch-all 'dustbin' diagnosis of IBS.

Perhaps you have been struggling with digestive symptoms for some time or have recently received an IBS diagnosis. Maybe you have a friend or family member who is struggling with the condition. Whatever your reasons for picking up this book, I'll take you through everything you need to know about IBS, including:

- **How the digestive system works**, and the role that the brain and gut microbiome play in a healthy gut

- **The main symptoms and types of IBS** – and the red-flag symptoms you should never ignore

- **How to get the most out of your medical appointments**

- **Everything you've ever wanted to know about bowel movements** – but have been too embarrassed to ask.

And, crucially, we'll be looking at strategies showing you how to successfully manage your symptoms in order to achieve that all-important quality of life, including medication, diet, exercise and psychological therapies.

IBS can be a very isolating syndrome, but you are certainly not alone. In fact IBS is a proverbial iceberg condition, whereby the majority of people with IBS symptoms haven't even been diagnosed yet. That's why you'll be reading stories from patients of all ages and symptoms who have regained control of their lives, using the right treatment.

It really is possible to have a happy, fulfilling life with IBS, and I'll show you how. This book is about taking a deeper look at IBS, so that you can get to know your own body better and take charge of your health and treatment. Self-empowerment and acceptance of this diagnosis go a long way towards improved quality of life.

1. Inside Our Digestive System, and Understanding IBS

What does a 'normal' digestive system look like?

Often patients will say to me, 'I feel I am not digesting my food properly' or 'I feel like there's something wrong with my gut.' This feeling can mean anything from nausea to heartburn, to seeing food remnants in one's stool.

Before we look at IBS in more detail, it is worth taking a step back to understand the basics of our digestive system. Having a greater knowledge of this intricate process will help you understand the reasons why parts of the process can go awry and trigger IBS symptoms. In this chapter I will also outline what IBS is, and show why it is very much a 'real' diagnosis. We'll also look at advances in our knowledge about IBS over the last decade and why this is a very exciting time for IBS and other symptom-based syndromes.

How the digestion system works

Our bodies rely on the food we eat to give us energy, help our growth and for repair.

Digestion is the process that helps us extract what we

need from food. Large insoluble food molecules are broken down into smaller water-soluble molecules so that they can be absorbed into the bloodstream more easily. Digestion is both mechanical and chemical: mechanical in the sense that food is broken down by muscular contractions in the gastrointestinal (GI) tract, and chemical because enzymes break down food into small molecules that the body can use.

This process isn't down to just one organ, but to a series of organs working together. I became a gastroenterologist because I was fascinated by the variety of organs within

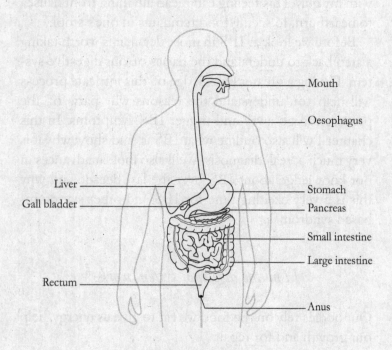

The digestive system

the GI tract, the multitude of processes that occur within each organ and the innate connection to our brain – something we have been coming to fully understand only in recent years.

What is the digestive system?

Our digestive system is an extremely complex, uniquely designed and intricate combination of the GI tract and our liver, pancreas and gall bladder. Think of it as the engine room of the body, which houses our 'second brain' (see page 14).

The GI tract is a lengthy system of organs joined as a long, twisting tube from the mouth to the anus. This starts at the mouth and follows through the oesophagus, stomach, small intestine (or small bowel), large intestine (also known as the large bowel or colon) to the rectum and anus, where stool is excreted or passed out of the body.

Our gut microbiome – which is made up of trillions of microorganisms, including bacteria, viruses and parasites in our GI tract (see Chapter 6) – also aids digestion. The brain and the nerves to the gut are closely involved in digestion as well, as is the blood supply to the gut.

The other organs that make up the digestive system are our liver, pancreas and gall bladder. All the organs of our digestive system, along with hormones, nerves, bacteria and blood supply, work closely in sync to enable the daily digestion of the foods and liquids we ingest and drink to produce nutrients that are used for the body's energy, growth and cell repair.

Starting from the top, let's look at the twists and turns of the digestive system and the key role that each part plays. It's on average a 9-m (30-ft) journey from beginning to end.

- **Mouth**: Digestion starts here, at the first bite of a meal. We chew to break down our food into smaller pieces so that it is easier to digest, and food is mixed with saliva to start the process of digestion. When you swallow, the tongue pushes food into the throat. A small flap called the epiglottis folds over our windpipe to protect it and prevent choking, and the food passes into the oesophagus.

- **Oesophagus**: This is a muscular tube extending from the pharynx/throat to the stomach. The brain sends signals to the muscles of the oesophagus to allow food to pass through in a series of wave-like muscle contractions known as peristalsis. Food moves down to the lower oesophageal sphincter, a ring-like muscle that relaxes, opens and lets food pass into the stomach. This acts as a valve that prevents food passing back up into the oesophagus.

- **Stomach**: This is a large hollow organ with strong and efficient muscular walls. A series of muscular contractions (known as trituration) mix and grind the food particles into smaller and smaller pieces, aided by secreted acid and powerful enzymes that continue breaking down the food. By the time food is ready to exit the stomach, it is the consistency of a liquid or paste, called chyme. This passes through another muscular sphincter, known as the pylorus, into the small intestine.

- **Small intestine (or small bowel):** A long tube lying centrally in the abdomen more than about 7m (23 ft) long, the small intestine is the longest part of the GI tract. It is made up of three segments: the duodenum, the jejunum and the ileum.

  The duodenum continues the process of breaking down food, utilizing enzymes released by the pancreas and bile from the liver, which is stored in the gall bladder. Bile is a liquid that enables the digestion of fats and eliminates waste products from the blood.

  The jejunum and ileum are mainly responsible for the absorption of nutrients into the bloodstream. The muscles of the small intestine mix food with the digestive juices and propel the mixture forward for further digestion. As peristalsis continues, the remaining waste products of the digestive process move into the large intestine.

- **Large intestine (large bowel or colon):** This is a 1.8-m (6-ft)-long muscular tube where waste left over from the digestive process (known as faeces or stool) is passed through by peristalsis. Stool is

9

made up of undigested parts of food, fluid, bacteria and older cells from the lining of the GI tract. This starts as a liquid, which becomes solidified as water is removed from the stool as it passes through the colon. The bacteria serve useful functions, such as synthesizing various vitamins, processing waste products and food particles and protecting against harmful bacteria.

- **Rectum**: Latin for 'straight', the rectum is located at the lower end of the large intestine, where stool is stored. The rectum lets us know there is stool to be evacuated and holds it until it is appropriate to have a bowel movement.

- **Anus**: The anus is the last part of the GI tract and is a complex structure made up of pelvic-floor muscles and two anal sphincters (internal and external muscles).

  The lining of the upper anus is programmed to detect rectal contents and its form – liquid, gas or solid. The pelvic-floor muscles create an angle between the rectum and the anus that stops stool from coming, while the anal sphincters control the stool. For example, the internal sphincter stops us having a bowel movement when we are asleep or otherwise unaware of the presence of stool. Nerve sensors in the internal sphincter send messages to the brain, which decides if it's an optimal time for a bowel movement.

If it is, the sphincter muscles relax and the rectum contracts, allowing a bowel movement. If the brain decides it isn't the right time, the external sphincter contracts and the urge to have a bowel movement is suppressed and the stool is kept in until we can get to the toilet.

The other organs playing a vital role in digestion are:

- **Pancreas**: An oblong-shaped gland in the upper midline of the abdomen, the pancreas secretes enzymes into the small intestine. These enzymes serve to break down proteins, fat and carbohydrates in the food we eat.

- **Liver**: This is a large, solid organ on the right-hand side of the abdomen under the ribs. Two of its main functions for the digestive system are to make and secrete bile and to cleanse and detoxify the blood coming from the small intestine containing absorbed nutrients.

- **Gall bladder**: This is a pear-shaped sac sitting just under the liver, which stores bile made in the liver. The gall bladder contracts at mealtimes to expel bile into the small intestine to allow for nutrient absorption in the small intestine.

Now that we have an understanding of how the GI tract and the wider digestive system work, let's look at the common symptoms of IBS.

What is IBS?

IBS involves episodes of abdominal pain and changes to the pattern of bowel movements. It is a syndrome, and so it is a collection of associated symptoms, as opposed to a specific disease. Symptoms vary from person to person in both type and severity. However, in addition to abdominal pain, they may include:

- Diarrhoea

- Constipation

- Distension

- Straining during a bowel movement

- A sensation of incomplete bowel-emptying

- Urge to visit the bathroom suddenly

- Mucus seen with the stools

- Symptoms made worse by eating.

Bloating is another commonly reported symptom, but it is not mandatory for the diagnosis of IBS.

The Bristol Stool Chart is a medical guide designed to classify stool form. Health professionals will often refer to this chart when discussing a diagnosis of IBS, and it is also a helpful tool for you to refer to when discussing symptoms with your doctor. Every person will have slightly different stool form, which will change, depending on diet.

Type 1		Separate hard lumps, like nuts (hard to pass)
Type 2		Sausage-shaped but lumpy
Type 3		Like a sausage but with cracks on its surface
Type 4		Like a sausage or snake, smooth and soft
Type 5		Soft blobs with clear-cut edges (passed easily)
Type 6		Fluffy pieces with ragged edges, a mushy stool
Type 7		Watery, no solid pieces, **Entirely liquid**

S. J. Lewis, K. W. Heaton (1997), 'Stool form scale as a useful guide to intestinal transit time', Scandinavian Journal of Gastroenterology (32), pp. 920–24

Normal stools (Types 3 and 4 on the chart) are soft and easy to pass. The harder stools (Types 1 and 2) usually indicate constipation, while Types 5, 6 and 7 may indicate diarrhoea.

IBS diagnosis

There are some risk factors that can increase your likelihood of developing IBS, such as diet, an infection like gastroenteritis, anxiety, stress or depression, and even past childhood trauma. We'll go into more detail about these risk factors in the next chapter.

However, IBS isn't merely about what is going on inside our gut. The biggest step change in the diagnosis of IBS in recent years has been in our understanding of what is known as the gut–brain axis. This is the interaction between the central nervous system (CNS) and the enteric – or gut – nervous system (ENS), which is known as our 'second brain'. Our main brain and gut are hardwired to communicate with each other, and when a glitch occurs in the system, it can lead to the troublesome symptoms of IBS. I have dedicated a whole chapter to this exciting area (see Chapter 3), and as we deepen our understanding of how it impacts upon IBS, it is hoped that it will lead to new treatments.

Why it may be difficult
to receive a proper diagnosis

Sadly, studies show it can take up to four years on average for people with IBS to be diagnosed. In fact it is not uncommon for my patients to have consulted three or four doctors before they see me.

Because IBS is a disorder of function (the way the GI tract works), rather than a structural or biological cause, blood tests, stool examinations, imaging scans and more invasive camera investigations, such as endoscopy or colonoscopy (see page 63), can all return 'normal' results. Historically, patients with functional symptoms (that is, symptoms with no physical cause) have traditionally been given short shrift as a result: they will have their symptoms investigated, but when the tests come back as normal, they are given little help to better understand or manage their condition.

Laura, 22

Law graduate Laura has always had what she describes as a sensitive tummy. As a child she remembers being fed prunes to help her go to the bathroom. At university she relied on multiple cups of coffee and cigarettes to keep her 'regular'. She sought help from her family doctor, who diagnosed IBS and told her to use over-the-counter medicine to relieve stomach cramps and to add extra fibre to her diet to help with regular bowel movements.

Although she followed her doctor's advice, Laura found these measures actually made her symptoms worse and instead turned to herbal teas. The past year had been a particularly stressful one, with university exams, and Laura had had constant stomach ache. Her stools had become harder and more difficult to pass, and she was now managing to go to the toilet only twice per week; and even then she only produced what she referred to as 'rabbit droppings'.

Laura started a new job at a law firm, where she had to wear a suit every day. But because her stomach would swell immediately after eating, she was afraid to eat during work hours in case her colleagues and clients would notice it. The pain and embarrassment were severely affecting her daily life, and she felt at a loss concerning how to manage her symptoms.

When Laura came to see me, we discussed her daily routine. She told me how she often felt the need to go to the toilet, but was too busy to go. We also reviewed her food intake, which had been whittled down to shop-bought salads, eaten on the run, and stodgy dinners, as she was ravenous by the evening. She was bloated, uncomfortable and wasn't sleeping well.

Interestingly Laura also revealed that she had three sisters who also had stomach problems, and her mum and aunt suffered from constipation. In the course of our conversation, suddenly Laura could see the link in similar symptoms within the family.

We discussed some over-the-counter treatment options, which she tried for a few months. I also advised her to stop her insoluble fibre intake, as this often makes for difficult symptoms in IBS patients. Over a number of months Laura gradually started to feel better. Instead of ignoring the urge to go to the toilet, she now goes when her body tells her to. And she is drinking more water, eating more regularly (particularly fruit) and has had a slow but consistent reduction in her symptoms.

Why a full discussion about symptoms is crucial

IBS is what is known as a 'positive diagnosis' – that is, a diagnosis based on discussion of symptoms, a full medical history and examination.

Some tests may still be needed to rule out other causes completely. These tests include a blood test to check for problems such as coeliac disease or thyroid disease, as the symptoms can overlap. A stool sample is also frequently required, to check for infection and inflammatory bowel disease.

How IBS is diagnosed

The Rome Foundation, founded in the 1980s, is an association of global experts focused on improving the diagnosis and treatments for functional GI disorders. The foundation has helped to legitimate these disorders, and central to this is the development of criteria for healthcare professionals to refer to when diagnosing disorders such as IBS – these are known as the Rome Criteria. The diagnostic criteria have been revised over time as more has become known about IBS. Now in their fourth iteration, the Rome IV Criteria were published in 2016.

The Rome IV Criteria should be based on a thorough medical history and define IBS as:

- **Recurrent abdominal pain** for on average at least one day per week in the last three months, associated with **two or more** of the following:

- Defecation symptoms getting better, or worse

- A change in the frequency of stool

- A change in the form (appearance) of stool.

It also states that symptoms should have started at least six months ago. Doctors should be able to make a diagnosis of IBS using the Rome IV Criteria and a limited number of tests alone. If any red-flag symptoms are reported – such as bleeding or sudden weight loss, which could suggest another problem – then (and only then) would more invasive investigations be requested.

Another key change in the Rome IV Criteria is that functional GI-tract disorders are now known as 'disorders of gut–brain interaction' (DGBI) to reflect our deepening understanding of the role of the gut–brain axis. Functional symptoms are experiences perceived by patients as being different from normal, and the consistent association of various symptoms makes up a syndrome. Although the word 'functional' has long been used medically, in more recent years there has been a decision to eliminate this term, because of its stigmatizing potential. Moreover, understanding the newer underlying mechanisms of IBS enables its more meaningful classification as a DGBI.

We are at an exciting time in our understanding of IBS: research efforts are concentrated on identifying a biological marker found in blood, stool or other tissues that will positively indicate the diagnosis of IBS. Research is ongoing and our understanding of IBS is evolving, paving the way for potential treatments to improve symptoms and the quality of life of IBS patients.

Subtypes of IBS

IBS is divided into the following subtypes, based on the dominant symptoms that a person experiences. These subtypes are known as:

- IBS-C where the patient will predominantly suffer from constipation
- IBS-D where the patient will predominantly suffer from diarrhoea
- IBS-M: 'mixed', that is, the patient can experience both types of bowel habits
- IBS unclassified: patients meet the diagnostic criteria for IBS, but cannot be

accurately categorized into one of the other subtypes given above.

The problem with these subtypes, however, is that they don't reflect the fact that symptoms do not always remain the same and, indeed, do change over time. We are now moving towards putting less emphasis on subclassification of symptoms, and instead carrying out a thorough clinical evaluation of what is causing the primary symptoms. I believe this is a positive step forward, as it will help us to tailor treatments to the individual and improve patient satisfaction and quality of life.

The impact of IBS and why it needs to be taken seriously

Both the diagnosis and management of IBS are fraught with difficulty and despair, for both patients and physicians alike.

Although IBS is not a 'disease', it can be extremely distressing. For the sufferer, these symptoms are very real. The majority of IBS sufferers manage their symptoms without seeking medical care, but those with moderate to severe symptoms who seek help from their family doctors and are eventually referred to specialist gastroenterologists are experiencing a markedly reduced quality of life.

One study showed that a majority of patients would give up 10–15 years of life expectancy for an instant cure for their condition.[1] Another study found that some patients with IBS would accept a risk of sudden death of 1 per cent, if a hypothetical medication could cure their symptoms.[2] These astonishing findings underline why we need to take IBS seriously, and that starts with the doctor–patient relationship.

Things are improving, but at times I have been surprised and exasperated by the apparent lack of interest in IBS among some of my fellow hospital doctors. It would appear that IBS doesn't have the same 'sexiness factor' as cancer or inflammatory bowel disease, both of which may present with the same symptoms.

Historically there has been prejudice towards IBS within the medical profession, stemming from a wrongly-held general bias about 'organic' versus 'functional' diagnoses. Just because IBS isn't explained with a simple test, that doesn't make it any less worthy of a doctor's time. Over the years my patients have recounted some distressing conversations when they have tried to seek help. 'It's all in your head,' one man was told. 'You're a woman and under stress – you only have IBS' was the verdict to another patient. And 'You need to see a psychiatrist.'

Many physicians will admit to feeling frustrated with the uncertain diagnosis and lack of treatment options for IBS. Fortunately we are learning so much more about IBS, especially as gut-microbiome research is rapidly expanding. We also have far more in our treatment armoury than in years gone by.

Increasingly, as hospital doctors, we are challenged by time pressures to see more patients in shorter visits, thus eroding the patient–provider relationship. Evidence shows that many patients with IBS are unhappy with their care: there are feelings of irritation, a sense of isolation and, sadly, dissatisfaction with their physicians, with the information received and with the healthcare system in general.

A good, supportive doctor–patient relationship can be as healing as treatment itself. Patients need, and deserve, to feel heard as well as having their symptoms validated. And a positive relationship has multiple benefits for patients and doctors alike. Both will feel more satisfied with a continuous rapport, and patients are more likely to stick to their medication and treatment plans.

Much of our medical training focuses on treating the disease, but many doctors relish treating the patient holistically by looking at their symptoms and individual experiences. Undoubtedly simply promoting a trusting relationship between a doctor and patient will lead to more effective treatment of IBS.

The financial and human impact of IBS

Investigating and treating IBS is costly: annual costs in the UK alone are estimated to be between £45 million and £200 million, and in the US between $1.5 billion and $10 billion per year. This is excluding prescription and over-the-counter medication costs.

One review estimated that the annual costs for treatment and care per IBS patient averaged between £90 and £316 in the UK; between $742 and $7,547 in the US; €567 and

€862 in France; $259 CAD in Canada; €791 in Germany; and $92 in Iran.[3] There are, of course, other indirect costs to consider, as patients with IBS often find it difficult to work due to their symptoms. Both absenteeism (needing to take time off work) and presenteeism (at work, but struggling to perform at one's best) are at play here. Studies in Europe and Canada suggest that anywhere between 5 and 50 per cent of people with IBS require some time off work, due to their symptoms. Yet to fully understand the full financial impact of IBS, further research is needed on the use of sickness and disability benefits, and on the impact upon families as a whole.

2. IBS Risk Factors

Before getting a diagnosis of IBS, many patients spend a lot of time trying to pinpoint the cause of their symptoms. 'Is it something I have eaten – and do I need to exclude something from my diet?', 'Why me?', 'How come this is happening to me now?' are some of the common questions that patients will ask me.

Sadly, with IBS the answer is not always clear-cut, and we will have to look back over many months, if not years, to try to understand what has affected the gut adversely. Despite several decades of research into IBS, in all honesty we still do not fully understand this disorder and all of its underlying mechanisms. But what we do know is that IBS appears to be a result of a mix of individual inherent and external factors.

Risk factors and crucial concepts

In this chapter I will be taking you through the risk factors or events that can make someone more likely to develop IBS, from our genes and our diet through to antibiotics, stress and even past bouts of infections such as gastroenteritis. I will also be introducing you to the gut microbiome, which is transforming how we think about, and treat, IBS.

Risk factor 1: does IBS run in families?

While we are still in the infancy of our understanding of the genetic associations of IBS, it does occur more often in some families than would be expected within the general population. This is known as familial clustering. As with Rachel (see the case study on page 28), when I discuss family medical history with my patients, they often reveal that they have siblings or other close relatives who also suffer from 'stomach issues' or 'bowel or tummy troubles'.

One study suggests that 48 per cent of individuals with IBS have a first-degree relative with the syndrome. Some studies have shown an increased risk of IBS in identical twins while other studies have not, suggesting that environmental factors have a part to play in the prevalence in families. Families will share the same childhood experiences and environmental and dietary exposures.

It is hoped that advances in genomics – the study of the body's genes, their functions and their influence on the growth, development and working of the body – will tell us more about the role of genetics in IBS in the future.

Risk factor 2: diet

IBS is intricately linked to our diet. Dietary triggers for IBS symptoms include the high fat and sugar intake that is typical of Western diets, while Eastern cultures report more IBS in parallel with an increase in Westernization of their diets.

An important part of the diagnostic pathway is excluding coeliac disease (pronounced 'see-lee-ac'), where the body reacts to gluten – a protein found in grains, including wheat, rye, spelt and barley. Coeliac disease is common, affecting about 1 in 100 people, and many symptoms overlap with IBS, such as bloating, abdominal pain and diarrhoea. It is crucial that a correct diagnosis is made: in coeliac disease the immune system attacks the tissues in the gut when gluten is eaten. This damages the small intestine and affects the absorption of vital vitamins and minerals, leading to potential long-term complications, include osteoporosis, anaemia and an increased risk of cancers such as small-bowel cancer and lymphoma. To reduce symptoms and complications it is imperative that a strict, lifelong gluten-free diet is adhered to.

Other than coeliac disease, I always stress to my patients that it is unlikely we will find a specific dietary element that causes IBS. But over the last decade I am increasingly seeing a pattern of patients embarking on painstaking exclusion diets before they come to see me. And people aren't only cutting out gluten. Lactose intolerance – where the body is unable to digest the sugar lactose, found in milk and other dairy products – is another area of concern for many patients. Several patients I have seen in recent years have already self-diagnosed lactose intolerance and will have completely excluded dairy from their diet, with variable results.

While it is possible to have both coeliac disease and

lactose intolerance alongside IBS, a true food allergy only affects approximately 1 per cent of adult patients, and so finding a single dietary element causing IBS symptoms is unusual.

Please don't embark on significantly restricted diets before seeking medical advice. Restricting foods from your diet risks increasing anxiety, alters your microbiome and can affect the severity of your gut symptoms. A balanced diet is a complex thing, and the wholesale cutting out of entire food groups can have far-reaching effects beyond our digestive system.

Why gluten-free isn't necessarily better for you

In the UK the market for gluten-free foods has soared by 43 per cent, from £470 million in 2015 to a staggering £673 million in 2020. This figure underscores the shift in gluten-free approach away from medical necessity to mainstream diet.

Surveys have shown that 23 per cent of people buy gluten-free food despite not having coeliac disease. Why? This is partly due to the belief that gluten-free products are somehow 'healthier'. But gluten-free doesn't automatically mean something is better for you. In fact most gluten-free snacks are significantly higher in fats, sugars and have the same calorie content as normal comparable snacks – not to mention being more expensive.

The message is clear: if you have a diagnosis of coeliac disease, then a gluten-free diet is a lifesaving must. If you don't, give the 'free-from' aisles in the supermarket a miss.

Risk factor 3: disruption to the gut microbiome

The microbiome is the collective name given to the trillions of organisms such as bacteria, viruses and fungi that are living and thriving in our bodies. The overwhelming majority of these organisms are found within our gut, and thanks to an explosion of research over the last fifteen years, we know that the gut microbiome plays a hugely important role in general health, from metabolism and immune function to disease prevention.

There is also growing evidence that when this delicately balanced microbiome is disrupted – from factors such as infection or broad-spectrum antibiotic use – a person may be more susceptible to IBS. We will be delving into the gut microbiome in much more detail a bit later in the book (see Chapter 6).

Rachel, 35

Rachel experienced symptoms of diarrhoea, or soft, unformed stools, for about three months. Her abdomen felt uncomfortable most of the time and her diet was very restrictive, consisting of just fish, rice and boiled vegetables. She had lost a little bit of weight in recent months, noting that her jeans felt looser.

A visit to her family doctor resulted in a few stool samples being taken, but the tests came back as 'normal'. Rachel didn't find the appointments productive and so she didn't go back. She came to see me because her symptoms were not improving; in fact she no longer socialized because she was so worried that she would need the bathroom when she was out.

We talked through her medical history, which included panic attacks in a previous job, but Rachel said she was in a new role and was doing well. We discussed her family's medical history and she mentioned that her twin sister suffered from nausea and heartburn. I also asked about any recent travel, and Rachel recalled a gap year in Tanzania thirteen years previously when she was struck down with a nasty bout of food poisoning. She was admitted to hospital and required IV fluids and possibly antibiotics. Since then, Rachel had used senna teas on and off to help with constipation.

I requested some blood tests, including one that tests for antibodies usually present in people with coeliac disease. All were normal. I examined her abdomen; it was tender and quite bloated. We discussed Rachel's bowel habits further, and she often felt the need to go to the bathroom without any result.

In her case, the key was normal investigations and the

realization that the gastroenteritis episode thirteen years earlier was the significant trigger. I diagnosed Rachel with post-infectious IBS, which had been present in a milder form since the food poisoning.

After a trial of a less restrictive diet, along with soluble-fibre intake and a course of probiotics, Rachel's softer stools normalized. She is working on maintaining a more varied diet, and I am happy to say is managing her symptoms very well.

Risk factor 4: post-infectious IBS (known as PI-IBS)

This is a type of IBS triggered by an infection in the GI tract such as gastroenteritis. The link was first made during the Second World War, when soldiers returning to the UK who had suffered from bacterial dysentery while overseas went on to develop IBS-type symptoms.

During an infection like gastroenteritis, our body produces an immune response to the infection, causing the gut to become inflamed. For most of us, a nasty bout of infection will have us laid low for a couple of days, but we will regain full health soon afterwards. However, about one in ten patients with an acute gut infection will go on to develop PI-IBS, and the risk is increased in people who are prescribed antibiotics during the gut infection.

PI-IBS is mainly linked to infections caused by bacteria such as campylobacter, salmonella and shigella, but has been associated also with a parasite called giardia. Women tend to be affected more than men, with one study suggesting women are four times more likely to develop PI-IBS.[1]

The exact cause is not known, but it is thought that there is a delay in the body switching off the immune response, leaving the gut inflamed. In addition, the infection can damage nerve endings in the gut, affecting gut motility and sensation.

As our case study of Rachel shows, I find that this is a link that doesn't tend to be at the forefront of a patient's mind. But by digging a little deeper during a consultation, the patient may recall a long-forgotten bout of food poisoning or gastroenteritis while on holiday.

Risk factor 5: stress, anxiety and depression

Stress, anxiety and depression are closely associated with IBS and may make symptoms worse. Anxiety symptoms are seen in 39 per cent of patients with IBS, and depressive symptoms in 29 per cent. These issues may pre-date or be a consequence of IBS and are an example of the gut–brain axis in action.

The interactions of the gut–brain work both ways. Our moods and thought processes can affect our gut function, such as when nerves before an important event trigger nausea or diarrhoea. Similarly, our gut can trigger brain responses: think about how you react when you urgently need to visit a toilet – you might feel anxious, sweat and even experience palpitations. It is believed that gut-microbiome alterations may feed back into the brain and affect psychological well-being. Similarly, the brain has been shown to affect gut sensitivity and motility, and to trigger symptoms of IBS such as altered bowel habits and abdominal pain.

Studies show that not only are people with anxiety and depression at increased risk of developing IBS, but those who already have an IBS diagnosis show a significant increase in anxiety and depression when they are followed up.

Another factor at play is serotonin – a neurochemical that assists the transmission of signals between nerves. This chemical exists in the brain and helps to regulate mood, but significantly is present in the gut too. Serotonin can affect gut motility (the way the gut moves) and physiology (how the gut interacts with other bodily systems like the immune system).

Recent advances in the treatment of IBS include therapies that help to regulate serotonin levels and activity. For example, in IBS with constipation, the aim is to stimulate serotonin receptors in the gut, particularly a serotonin type-4 receptor (known as 5-HT4), which helps promote peristalsis and accelerate the movement of stools through the gut. It is hoped that understanding more about these processes will provide future treatment options, and we may even reach a stage one day in the future where we look at the prevention of IBS, rather than simply managing the symptoms.

Risk factor 6: past antibiotic use

Most of us will have been prescribed and taken antibiotics at some point in our lives. However, these days there is growing awareness that not all infections need antibiotic treatment, and we need to avoid the knee-jerk response to take antibiotics. This is mostly to prevent antibiotic resistance, where bacteria learn to change and outwit the antibiotic treatment. Bacterial resistance is increasing worldwide at an alarming rate. A growing number of infections – such as pneumonia, tuberculosis, gonorrhoea and salmonellosis (caused by the salmonella bacterium) – are becoming harder to treat as the antibiotics used to combat them become less effective. This leads to higher medical costs, prolonged hospital stays and increased death rates, according to the World Health Organization, which deems antibiotic resistance to be one of the biggest threats to global health today.

As we have seen with the COVID-19 pandemic, behavioural changes are paramount. This is to reduce the spread of infection, through hand-washing, practising safer hygiene techniques and meticulous food-handling.

Of course there are many instances where antibiotics are necessary and even lifesaving. But antibiotic treatment and gut-related side-effects often go hand-in-hand, probably due to the antibiotics disrupting the microbiome. It is widely confirmed that more than 75 per cent of people with IBS will have used antibiotics in the previous twelve months.

Risk factor 7: early life experiences

Our gut health comes into play from the day we are born. Our gut microbiome at birth is of low diversity, but by the time we reach two years of age it has grown in complexity and diversity and is akin to the gut microbiome seen in adults. So the first year or so of life is crucial to the development of a healthy microbiome. For example, breast milk is the main influencing factor in the composition of the microbiome.

There are contradictory studies looking at socioeconomic status and the risk for IBS. It appears that lower-income families and those living in crowded and unhygienic conditions have a higher risk of developing IBS. This may be related to a greater risk of developing gastroenteritis or needing antibiotic treatments. But at the same time there is also risk of IBS in more affluent families, which some have put down to the strain of greater emphasis on academic achievement, which could lead to stress and anxiety and affect an individual's coping mechanisms.

Interestingly, research has also found an increased risk of developing IBS in people who were subjected to emotional, sexual and/or psychological abuse in childhood. Parents with a history of IBS, mental illness, anxiety and/or depression, substance abuse and negative parenting styles transmit an increased risk of IBS to their children. On the flipside, other studies have shown a reduced risk of IBS where subjects have enjoyed warm, caring and supportive relationships in early childhood.

3. The Gut–Brain Axis Explained

Have you ever felt butterflies in your stomach ahead of a job interview or found yourself rushing to the toilet just before an important occasion? Or maybe you've gone with your 'gut instinct' when faced with a difficult decision?

Whether we realize it or not, our brain and our gut are intrinsically linked. Information is constantly running back and forth between the two in a complex network of nerve cells, or neurons.

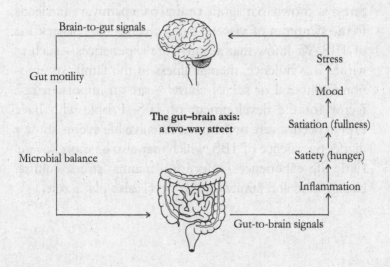

Brain-to-gut signals

Gut motility

Microbial balance

The gut–brain axis:
a two-way street

Stress

Mood

Satiation (fullness)

Satiety (hunger)

Inflammation

Gut-to-brain signals

There are between 200 and 600 million neurons lining the gut that form part of the enteric nervous system (ENS). This is connected to our brain – the central nervous system (CNS) – via the vagus nerve, which runs from the brainstem down to the abdomen.

The neurons found in our gut are extremely complex and very closely mirror the nerves in our brain, in terms of their size and function. In fact about 90 per cent of the neurotransmitters (chemical messengers) that regulate our mood, such as serotonin and dopamine, are made in the gut. So perhaps it is unsurprising that the ENS is known as the 'second brain'. As an example, high serotonin levels are seen in patients with diarrhoea-predominant IBS, while low levels of serotonin are associated with constipation-predominant IBS.

This close relationship explains why we might experience a nervous butterfly-stomach or pre-exam diarrhoea. Stress is known to magnify central pain pathways and leads to the symptom of visceral pain, which is the cornerstone of IBS. We know that negative life experiences – such as witnessing violence, mental illness in the family or emotional, physical or sexual abuse[1] – are an important risk factor for the development of IBS. People who have experienced severe or frequent negative life events show a higher prevalence of IBS, which may also be more severe. Early life experiences, infections, trauma, stress, cultural background and family support levels also play a role.

What does the gut–brain axis have to do with IBS?

The relatively recent acceptance of the gut–brain axis has helped deepen our understanding of IBS for both patients and doctors alike. We know that the gut–brain axis includes the ENS and the CNS, but it also involves:

- **The neuroendocrine immune system**, which regulates hormones and the immune system

- **The hypothalamic–pituitary–adrenal (HPA) axis**: these three glands help to regulate metabolism, mood, stress response, energy and immunity

- **The autonomic nervous system (ANS)**, which aids peristalsis – the automatic wave-like contractions to help food and waste move through the GI tract.

Imagine all these systems working together like a circuit board. This whole circuitry plays a crucial role in IBS by regulating gut motility, visceral sensitivity (pain sensitivity, common in people with IBS), stress responses and brain function.

How are the gut microbiome, the gut–brain axis and IBS connected?

As research has evolved over the last five years, IBS has been reclassified as a disease of a gut–brain axis dysregulation – in 2016 the Rome Foundation updated its definition of IBS to reflect this. The gut microbiome has garnered tremendous research interest in the last decade, starting in the US with the Human Microbiome Project, which ran from 2007 to 2016.

This US $157 million project enabled the study of the microbial communities that live in and on our bodies, and of the roles they play in human health and disease. It resulted in more than 650 scientific papers being published. Several other countries, including the UK, Germany, France, Canada and China, have also increased their investment and interest in this rapidly advancing field.

The gut microbiome is known to affect our metabolism, immunity, endocrine and neural processes, and thus to affect our health. We know of a newly discovered intimate association of our microbiome and disease processes: both general such as heart disease or diabetes, and gut conditions such as colorectal cancer and IBS.

The strongest evidence that these three entities – the microbiome, the gut–brain axis and IBS as a condition – are all interconnected is in the case of PI-IBS. As we now know, IBS can be triggered by a bout of gastroenteritis, whether bacterial, viral or parasitic.

We know that the gut microbiome (and any stool samples) has a different make-up and diversity in IBS patients compared to healthy patients. And low-grade gut inflammation appears to be present in many IBS patients, which we now think could be related to a damaged microbiome or dysbiosis (where the bacteria in the gut is unbalanced). Therefore therapies targeting the microbiome in IBS could be an effective approach. It has been shown that some IBS patients show a good response to non-absorbable antibiotics (such as rifaximin, which I will cover in more detail on page 108). I will also discuss prebiotic and probiotic options for symptom relief. Another emerging treatment option for IBS is faecal transplantation. Established as a treatment for *Clostridium difficile* (bacterial) infection, faecal transplantation is the transfer of healthy bacteria in a mixture of prepared, processed stool from a healthy donor to the intestine of a patient. However, for IBS it is a treatment that is still very much in its infancy and yet to be fully studied, given the risks of also transmitting ill health.

What the gut–brain axis connection could mean for future treatments

When it comes to the gut microbiome, we know that our gut bacteria can impact on our brains, as well as contribute to neurological and psychiatric disease, such as depression, Parkinson's disease, IBS, Alzheimer's disease and drug addiction. Studies have also shown that disturbances in the gut–brain axis drive the development of several gastro-intestinal diseases, including inflammatory bowel disease (IBD), such as ulcerative colitis and Crohn's disease. Indeed IBS and IBD can overlap in the same patient.

In up to half of IBS cases where gut symptoms appear first, there is a subsequent onset of mood and anxiety disorders. Does this mean that the gut is driving the brain manifestations? Some studies looking into the gut microbiome, intestinal inflammation and gut-related immune responses further suggest that the gut may drive alterations in the brain. Excitingly, if this finding is ultimately proven to be accurate, then reversing gastrointestinal dysfunction may be a potential treatment option in curing IBS of its associated psychological disorders. Therapies targeting the microbiome are an exciting and potential area of treatment in the future, but we are not quite there yet with our research. There are many gaps in our knowledge and full understanding of the dysbiotic microbiome in IBS and of the pathophysiological mechanisms to allow for safe and effective targeted therapies. We need to wait for further large-scale controlled trials of both existing and newer treatments to enhance our understanding in this new, rapidly changing field. It is probably within this arena that precision medicine tailored to differing IBS subtypes will emerge, and thereby pave the way for personalized medicine options.

As previously mentioned, the Rome IV Criteria – the worldwide gold standard in diagnosing IBS – now refers to it as a disorder of gut–brain interaction.

One key area for treatment comprises the links between IBS and psychiatric conditions. Research shows the most common mental-health conditions seen in people with IBS are anxiety disorders (the prevalence is about 30–50 per cent) and depression (70 per cent). Eating disorders are also seen, although these are less frequent. Another study has shown that catastrophizing, which is defined as expecting a negative outcome, is more common in IBS patients.

This important link plays a role in the selection of

potential treatments that are considered for IBS symptoms, particularly when other options such as medication have not had an effect. We will cover these therapies also in Chapter 8, but they include:

- Talking therapies such as psychotherapy and cognitive behavioural therapy (CBT)

- Gut-directed hypnotherapy

- Mindfulness-based therapy

- Relaxation therapy, such as deep breathing and visualization.

The IBS community is increasingly recognizing the potential in psychological therapies: a review by the World Gastroenterology Organisation found that CBT, hypnotherapy and psychodynamic therapy are effective in improving IBS symptoms. In addition, 2021 guidance on IBS management by the American College of Gastroenterology endorsed gut-directed psychotherapies alongside medical and dietary treatments for IBS patients.

Hypnotherapy

Far from the clichéd image of a watch being swung in front of a sleepy patient, gut-directed hypnotherapy is an evidence-based therapy that is specifically designed for people with GI disorders. The science of gut-directed hypnotherapy is still in its infancy, and the precise mechanism for how this relieves

IBS symptoms is not fully known. Several theories suggest effects might occur by:

- Reducing sensitivity to gut pain

- Relaxing the smooth muscle in the intestine

- Increasing motility (the speed of food moving through the gut)

- Reducing the psychological trait of somatization, which is body sensation-focused distress.

Australian researchers recently showed that hypnotherapy is an effective treatment for irritable bowel syndrome. The team from Monash University in Melbourne, Australia, showed that hypnotherapy was equal in effectiveness to their low-FODMAP diet for relieving symptoms of IBS such as bloating and abdominal pain (we'll be looking at the FODMAP diet in more detail on page 124).

How can it help me?

Gut-directed hypnotherapy looks to address any emotional or stress triggers that can exacerbate IBS symptoms, such as pain, constipation, diarrhoea or bloating. During hypnotherapy patients are eased into a deeply relaxed or hypnotic state, where they are better able to respond to positive suggestions to help certain behaviours or responses to pain.

There is a growing body of evidence about the benefits of gut-directed hypnotherapy. A 2019 study involving

350 people with IBS found that those who participated in individual or group gut-directed hypnotherapy sessions had better relief from symptoms compared to those who attended education sessions. Researchers also found that this effect lasted for nine months after the sessions ended.[2]

Gut-directed hypnotherapy can be delivered one-to-one or in a group setting. While the exact process varies between practitioners, the UK's National Council for Hypnotherapy states that sessions generally include:

- Visualization for the desired outcome when you are free of symptoms

- Processing any worries or fears that may be contributing to IBS

- Visualization and suggestions to decrease gut sensitivity and increase well-being

- Learning self-hypnosis

- An audio recording to use between sessions.[3]

How do I access it?

In the UK hypnotherapy is recommended as a therapy for IBS on the National Health Service (NHS), but availability may depend on where you live. Waiting times are extremely long, however. Although this may not be an accessible option for all people suffering from IBS, you may find it quicker to access help privately. When choosing a hypnotherapist, always check they are trained to deliver gut-directed hypnotherapy and are registered with a professional association, such as the National Council for Hypnotherapy in the UK (see Further Reading and Resources on page 177).

Cognitive behavioural therapy (CBT)

CBT is a talking therapy used for a variety of physical and mental-health issues and is an increasingly common treatment for IBS.

How can it help me?

CBT aims to help patients respond to challenges in a more positive way, by breaking them down into smaller parts. It centres on the concept that our thoughts, feelings, physical sensations and actions are interconnected, and that negative thoughts and feelings can trap us in a vicious cycle. Unlike psychotherapy, CBT focuses on the present and our response to situations. For example:

- **Situation**: You need to use the toilet while out for a meal with friends

- **Thought**: 'Everyone will notice if I am gone for a long time'

- **Feelings**: Anxiety, fear, embarrassment

- **Physical sensations**: Stomach pain

- **Behaviour**: You don't eat, to avoid having to use the toilet.

The aim of CBT is to help you recognize and unpick unhelpful feelings and behaviours and develop strategies so that you react to challenges in a more positive way. Studies have shown that CBT for IBS is highly effective in improving symptoms, quality of life and psychological distress, and these positive effects can be felt after the sessions have ended.[4]

How do I access it?

CBT is a very well-established treatment that is used worldwide, so speak to your medical team about how you can access it.

If you live in the UK, you can ask your family doctor to refer you to an NHS psychological-therapies service. You can self-refer too. However, waiting times may be long, so going private is another option. The British Association for Behavioural and Cognitive Psychotherapies has a list of accredited CBT therapists. Outside the UK, you can speak to your health provider about how to access talking therapies that are specifically aimed at helping people with IBS. There are other options available too. One study looked at self-administered CBT, which was found to be significantly more effective than an education intervention, and comparable to intensive clinic-based CBT in improving symptoms of IBS.[5]

Physical location is no longer a barrier to accessing digital

CBT, with apps such as Bold Health's Zemedy, which is a six-week CBT programme.[6] In addition, Mindset's Nerva IBS app is a six-week gut-directed hypnotherapy app.[7]

Mindfulness

Mindfulness is the practice of being 'in the moment' and paying attention to your thoughts, your surroundings and the sensations of your breathing and your body. With mindfulness, the aim is not to empty your mind of worries, but to notice them, acknowledge them and visualize them passing through.

How can it help me?

Mindfulness is increasingly being used with issues such as stress, anxiety, depression and insomnia. Evidence on its effectiveness for IBS is limited, but growing. A small study of fifty-three people with IBS found that they experienced fewer gastrointestinal symptoms after they participated in a mindfulness programme designed to reduce stress.[8]

How do I access it?

Mindfulness can be done alone at home, but there are some structured courses available on the NHS, so speak to your family doctor about them. As with CBT, waiting lists can be long and their availability varies. You could opt for paid, private sessions. The British Association of

Mindfulness-Based Approaches has a list of qualified mindfulness teachers.

In 1979 the Mindfulness-Based Stress Reduction Clinic at the University of Massachusetts Medical Center was started. By 2015 close to 80 per cent of US medical schools offered some element of mindfulness training. Since then research and education centres dedicated to mindfulness have proliferated, to the extent that almost all large universities in the US are affiliated with mindfulness centres – Harvard, Johns Hopkins and Stanford among others.

Is personalized treatment the future?

We are still in the infancy of our understanding of the gut–brain axis and the gut microbiome, but this is an exciting time for those in the field, and for people with IBS. I believe that in the coming years we will use our individual genome and microbiome-sequence signature to diagnose and devise personalized treatments for conditions such as IBS.

4. Alarm Symptoms: When Are My Symptoms Not Down to IBS?

We have now covered the common signs, symptoms and risk factors associated with IBS. But when do symptoms stop being simply IBS and become something else?

IBS symptoms may not always be what they seem. If you are feeling bloated, suffer from stomach cramps or your toilet habits are irregular, sometimes these symptoms might not be down to an IBS diagnosis, but could be your body trying to tell you that something else is amiss.

Several symptoms of IBS overlap with other conditions and diseases. Other symptoms raise concerns among us, as doctors. These are 'alarm symptoms' or 'red flags' – that is, symptoms that are not explained by IBS and warrant additional investigations to rule out another condition. In this chapter I will be taking you through the alarm symptoms that you should be on the lookout for, and what to do if you have already noticed them or go on to develop them in future.

IBS can coexist with other conditions: for example, about one in ten people with IBS will also suffer from coeliac disease, while people with inflammatory bowel disease (IBD) – an umbrella term for diseases such as Crohn's and ulcerative colitis – can also suffer from IBS

New onset of
IBS-like symptoms
at the age of 50 or older

Blood in the stools
(even with prior history
of haemorrhoids) or
black stools

Symptoms such as
pain or diarrhoea wake
you up in the night

Unintentional or unexplained
weight loss

A change in typical IBS symptoms,
such as new or different pain or
a change in bowel habits

Family history of other GI diseases,
such as cancer, IBD or coeliac disease

Blood tests revealing anaemia
or inflammation

The alarm symptoms you should never ignore

symptoms. But while the symptoms may be very similar, conditions like IBS, coeliac disease and IBD are very different and each requires a proper diagnosis and tailored treatment.

The key thing to remember is that *you* know your own body. With our busy lives, it can be all too easy to miss red flags and any changes. It is important not to panic: not all alarm symptoms are due to serious disease, but they are an indication that you should talk to your family doctor or gastroenterologist. It may be nothing, but if something doesn't feel quite right, then it is always worth asking for medical advice, even if only to put your mind at ease.

If it isn't IBS, then what could it be?

Below I have outlined some of the most common conditions and diseases to which alarm symptoms could be related.

Coeliac disease

This disease is much more common than previously thought. It is a digestive condition where sufferers have an adverse reaction to gluten, a protein found in wheat, rye and barley. When they eat gluten, the immune system attacks the tissues in the small intestine, causing damage and inflammation. The surface of a healthy small intestine is covered in millions of tiny finger-shaped growths called villi, which help to digest food effectively into the blood. But in coeliac disease, this damage and inflammation flatten the villi, so that the body is unable to absorb nutrients as well as it should.

Coeliac disease affects about one in 100 people in the UK, rising to about one in ten in those who have a close family member with the disease. Additional risk factors may include having other autoimmune conditions, such as an underactive thyroid. If you are concerned that you might be coeliac, you can ask your doctor to check with a blood test, but you must be on a gluten-containing diet for this to be meaningful. Coeliac disease is often diagnosed in people without symptoms, or with headaches, skin rash or infertility, rather than in those with the typical symptoms listed below.

Classic signs and symptoms

- Diarrhoea due to malabsorption of nutrients; malabsorption may also mean that stools are foul-smelling, greasy or frothy because of a high fat content

- Abdominal pain

- Wind and bloating

- Indigestion

- Constipation.

How is it diagnosed?

Routine testing for coeliac disease is not recommended unless you have symptoms or an increased risk of developing the disease. If coeliac disease is suspected, then your family doctor can carry out two blood tests:

- Total immunoglobulin A (IgA)

- IgA Tissue Transglutaminase Antibody (usually called tTG)

These tests measure the number of antibodies that the body produces in response to eating gluten. If the tests show a high number of antibodies, then a referral to a gastroenterologist for a biopsy may be necessary to confirm the diagnosis. A biopsy is a short procedure where a thin, flexible tube called an endoscope will be inserted into your mouth and the small intestine, where a tiny sample of the lining of the small intestine is taken and examined for damage that is typical of coeliac disease.

Note: It is crucial that you carry on eating gluten ahead of blood tests and a biopsy to ensure an accurate result.

How is it treated?

It is important to say that coeliac disease is exactly that: a disease, not an allergy or an intolerance. Treatment involves a referral to a gastroenterologist (and possibly a dietician too) and cutting gluten out of the diet completely for life, to avoid symptoms. The long-term complications of coeliac disease due to malabsorption may include anaemia or vitamin deficiencies and even osteoporosis, as well as lymphoma and small-intestinal cancers.

Bile-acid malabsorption

As we saw in Chapter 1, bile is a liquid that is essential in helping the body to digest fats and eliminate waste products from the blood. Bile is released into the small intestine during the digestive process and then is for the most part reabsorbed, with only a small amount reaching the colon, where it is removed in the stools.

The problem arises when the body has trouble reabsorbing bile, so that more bile ends up in the colon than should do. This extra bile triggers the colon to release more water, speeding up the passage of waste through the colon. Think of it as being like when you get soap in your eyes: they water. In a similar way, bile acid irritates the tissue in the colon, causing it to 'water' too.

Symptoms

- Watery diarrhoea
- Bloating
- Cramps.

How is it diagnosed?

A SeHCAT (pronounced 'see-cat') scan is a two-stage test carried out in hospital to measure the body's ability to absorb bile. The first part involves taking a capsule containing an artificial bile-acid SeHCAT (75 Se-homocholic acid taurine), and then undergoing a scan a few hours later to measure how much of the capsule is absorbed. A second scan is performed seven days later to see how much of the tracer still remains. An absorption rate of above 15 per cent is classed as mild bile-acid malabsorption; 5–15 per cent indicates moderate; and below 5 per cent is severe.

How is it treated?

Bile-acid malabsorption is found in 30 per cent of IBS patients who experience diarrhoea. Although it is a lifelong, incurable condition, the good news is that it is very treatable. Medication called bile-acid sequestrants help reduce symptoms by binding to the bile acids in the small intestine, stopping them from irritating the large intestine.

Diet is also important: studies show that a low-fat diet can help to reduce symptoms,[1] and people who have the condition should aim to eat no more than 40g (1½ oz) of fat every day – to put that into perspective, a chocolate digestive has about 4g of fat, while a tablespoon of butter contains about 12g.

If you are battling with diarrhoea-predominant IBS, you should ask your doctor to refer you to a gastroenterologist for more help.

Inflammatory bowel disease (IBD)

Though IBS and IBD sound similar – and can often be used interchangeably in error – there is a crucial difference between the two terms. IBS is a syndrome (a collection of signs and symptoms) that, while often uncomfortable and painful, is not life-threatening. IBD, on the other hand, is a disease that can lead to life-threatening complications, if left untreated.

The term IBD is used to describe diseases that involve inflammation of the gut – the two scenarios being ulcerative colitis and Crohn's disease.

Ulcerative colitis is a disease where the immune system attacks healthy gut tissue, causing ulcers and inflammation in the lining of the large intestine (colon). It affects about 140,000 people in the UK.

Crohn's disease is another inflammatory condition that is slightly less common, affecting about 115,000 people in the UK. It can be found along the whole length of the gut, from the mouth to the anus, but most commonly develops in the ileum (the last part of the small intestine) or the colon.

Repeated periods of inflammation with IBD – known as flare-ups – can lead to a build-up of scar tissue in the gut and cause abscesses to develop. Up to half of all patients with Crohn's disease may develop fistulae, when inflammation spreads through the bowel wall, tunnelling through the layers of other tissues and potentially affecting other organs. This complicated problem will often require medication and surgery. Medical management is essential for reducing symptoms and the need for surgical intervention. *Note*: this is not seen in ulcerative colitis.

Symptoms

Key symptoms of both ulcerative colitis and Crohn's disease are:

- Recurrent diarrhoea, which may contain blood or mucus

- Abdominal pain

- Fatigue

- Loss of appetite

- Weight loss

- Anaemia (due to malabsorption of key nutrients).

How are ulcerative colitis and Crohn's disease diagnosed?

Unfortunately, it can take several years to make this diagnosis, as IBD is often initially mistaken for IBS. The average time to diagnosis can be up to seven years. It is also important to remember that IBS and IBD can coexist in the same patient.

The first step is usually blood tests, such as:

- **Full blood count:** A common blood test that looks at the three main types of blood cells – white blood cells, red blood cells and platelets – to give a picture of your general health.

- **Inflammatory marker tests**: These tests can detect raised levels of proteins in the blood that may be a sign of inflammation.

- **Ferritin and transferrin tests**: Ferritin and transferrin are proteins that help to store, use and transport iron around the body. Anaemia due to bleeding and/or malabsorption of nutrients can be a sign of IBD, and low levels of ferritin are indicative of iron-deficiency anaemia.

You should also be asked for a stool sample, to check for infection and distinguish IBD from IBS.

The next step would be a referral to a gastroenterologist for further tests or investigations to confirm the diagnosis. This can include an endoscopy and/or a colonoscopy (see page 63) to take a closer look at the digestive system using an endoscope; and a biopsy may be taken.

You may also have imaging tests, such as an MRI or CT scan of the abdomen, or capsule endoscopy, which enables a clever camera in pill form to assess the entire small intestine.

Treatment

Treatment for IBD will depend on how much of the gut is affected, and how severe the case is.

In **ulcerative colitis**, the aim of initial treatment is to reduce inflammation to give damaged tissue a chance to heal. The first line treatment is aminosalicylates, also known as 5-ASAs. If these alone do not work, patients may be prescribed corticosteroids, which are used for more severe cases but cannot be used long-term, due to serious side-effects such as weakening of the bones or cataracts. Other treatments include:

- **Immunosuppressants**: Medicines that work to suppress or calm the immune system to prevent flare-ups are commonly prescribed.

- **Biologic medicines**: These medicines reduce inflammation by targeting and blocking proteins that stimulate inflammation. Biologic medicines may be considered if other options are unsuccessful.

- **Surgery**: In severe cases that are affecting quality of life, surgery to remove the colon may be considered.

Most people with **Crohn's disease** will be prescribed steroids to help reduce inflammation. Other treatments include:

- **Immunosuppressants**: as above

- **Biologic medicines**: as above

- **Surgery**: The most common operation is a resection, where the inflamed section of the bowel is removed and the remaining healthy parts of the bowel are stitched together.

Ovarian cancer

Ovarian cancer is the eighth most commonly occurring cancer in women worldwide, with nearly 300,000 new cases in 2018.[2] It is much more common in women over fifty. It is often asymptomatic in the early stages, but may present with a wide variety of vague and non-specific symptoms, including the following:

- Bloating: abdominal distension or discomfort
- Pressure effects on the bladder and rectum
- Constipation
- Vaginal bleeding
- Indigestion and acid reflux
- Shortness of breath
- Tiredness
- Weight loss
- Early satiety – feeling full easily
- Needing to urinate more often.

Unfortunately, most cases are diagnosed at an advanced stage.

Your family doctor should arrange a blood test called a CA125 test. CA125 is a protein that is often found on the surface of some ovarian cancer cells, and a high level of CA125 in the blood can be a sign of ovarian cancer. Women should also be referred for an ultrasound scan, particularly if they are aged fifty or over.

Treatment will depend on the stage and severity of cancer, but may include surgery and chemotherapy, or targeted therapies to treat advanced cancer.

John, 42

John, a successful architect, was referred to me after complaining of a 'twinge' on the right side of his abdomen every time he bent down to tie his laces. He was the model of politeness and was most apologetic for seeking medical advice.

During our first consultation he was quick to say that, aside from the afore-mentioned twinge, he didn't have any pain, was generally healthy and exercised regularly. He had no past medical history of concern and was not taking any medication. He was a pescatarian (someone who doesn't eat meat, but does eat fish) and enjoyed his food. We also discussed his lifestyle and any stresses, and John said he had wondered if working longer hours had resulted in work-related stress. He was engaged to be married the next year, and his fiancée had noticed that he complained of his discomfort after running and visiting the gym.

John had no weight loss, and described normal bowel habits. His physical examination was normal, other than being very mildly tender in the right abdomen. Our initial investigations with bloods, stool tests, X-ray and abdominal ultrasound were normal, so we discussed a trial period of smaller meals, upping his water intake and taking an over-the-counter antispasmodic to suppress the twinge.

After trying these measures, John reported feeling lighter, but that the twinge hadn't gone away. I reassured him again and this time arranged a diet evaluation, where he tried a modified version of the low-FODMAP diet (a diet that aims to identify triggers of IBS symptoms, see Chapter 8). At our follow-up he again reported the same symptoms and said he preferred to be on a regular meal plan, as the low-FODMAP diet was too restrictive.

His 'twinge' had not changed and was neither worse nor better. Given John's upcoming wedding and his persistent symptoms, I recommended a colonoscopy, which is a camera test to investigate the large intestine. This showed a large, flat polyp in the right colon and several smaller polyps in the left side. I was able to remove all of these through the endoscope; they were pre-cancerous polyps, so John will need ongoing follow-ups over the coming years.

When we reviewed his family history, there was no incidence of cancer in his immediate family (the risk of developing bowel cancer may be higher if a first-degree relative, such as a parent, sibling or child, has had the disease), but a great-aunt at the age of sixty and a second cousin at the age of forty-five had been diagnosed with colorectal cancer.

Because of the polyps, John has a higher risk of colorectal cancer, but with regular colonoscopy appointments every three to five years we can prevent this devastating consequence in the future. I am pleased to say that the 'twinge' settled, and John felt relieved that his polyps were removed and that he now has a screening plan in place. Best of all, John and his fiancée had a fabulous summer wedding.

Colorectal cancer

Colorectal cancer (also known as bowel cancer) is the third most common cancer in men and the second most common cancer in women worldwide,[3] with more than 1.93 million new cases in 2020. There are very successful screening programmes for colorectal cancer to prevent this disease. Screening aims to identify people at higher risk of this cancer before they have developed symptoms.

Patient selection for screening programmes is based on age and risk factors. It has been shown to increase uptake if screening for several different cancers is addressed together. For example, your family doctor discusses cervical-cancer screening at the same time as mammography screening for breast cancer and colorectal cancer.

However, it is important to seek advice if you notice new or persistent bowel symptoms.

Symptoms

- Persistent blood in the stools

- Persistent change in bowel habit

- Persistent lower abdominal pain or discomfort triggered by eating; this may be accompanied by reduced appetite or significant weight loss.

How is it diagnosed?

A doctor will carry out a digital rectal examination to check the rectum, which is a quick process. Blood tests may be requested to check for iron deficiency, as bleeding can lead to anaemia. Stool tests can detect hidden blood in the poo.

To make a definitive diagnosis you should be referred to hospital for a colonoscopy investigation, which involves a thin, flexible tube called a colonoscope (with a small camera attached) being inserted into the rectum and up into the large bowel. A biopsy may be taken to check for cancer cells. Polyps can also be removed during this procedure.

If a diagnosis is made, further tests will be undertaken to see if it has spread, and the cancer will be graded, depending on how big it is and whether it has spread.

How is it treated?

Early diagnosis is crucial: when identified early, colorectal cancer is more likely to respond to treatment and to result in a higher probability of survival. Early diagnosis consists of three key components:

1. Being aware of symptoms that may indicate cancer, and of the importance of seeking medical advice if you are concerned

2. Access to medical clinical evaluation and diagnostic services

3. Timely referral to treatment services.

Treatment will depend on where the cancer is and how far it has spread, but the main treatments are:

- **Surgery**, where the cancerous section of bowel is removed – this is the most common treatment for bowel cancer

- **Chemotherapy and radiotherapy** may also be used to kill cancer cells.

5. Associated Conditions

When patients come to see me for the first time, the initial appointment is all about letting them talk through their medical history. This discussion has two key elements. First, it is about your doctor listening to you, as you describe your symptoms and their impact on your life, plus any past illnesses and family medical history. Second, your doctor needs to be asking the right questions. The sign on my office door may say 'gastroenterologist', but I make a point of asking patients about other non-GI symptoms that they may have.

Often patients will be surprised when I ask questions about pain elsewhere, such as headaches, fatigue or pelvic pain, because they have arrived expecting to talk only about their bowel habits, gas or bloating. But I will say to you now as I say to them: there is no 'right' or 'wrong' information, when it comes to your consultation. Looking at each organ or part of the body in isolation runs the risk of crucial details being missed, which is frustrating for patients and physicians alike.

Research and the experiences of my patients show that people with IBS tend to suffer from other functional conditions[1] – that is, something that won't show up in any one test or procedure. But just because a test comes back as normal, that doesn't mean there isn't a problem. This may then lead to the patient being told that 'Nothing is wrong with you' or that it is all in their head.

We have an impressive battery of diagnostic tests at our disposal, such as blood and stool tests, X-rays and scans designed to identify structural and organic problems, but none of these tests evaluate dysfunction, where the GI tract looks normal when examined, but doesn't work properly. Yet functional pain conditions, such as fibromyalgia, chronic pelvic pain, migraine, chronic fatigue syndrome and temporomandibular joint disorder, share many similarities, and they are common in people with IBS. For example, up to 30 per cent of those with IBS also suffer from headaches and migraine, adding to their burden of suffering and affecting their quality of life.

Questions asked during a consultation can also be important. Often these questions take the conversation in a new direction, and patients will reveal months or even years of symptoms they haven't ever spoken about before.

In this chapter we will be looking at these functional disorders that can be associated with IBS. It may be that you recognize some of the symptoms described here, and this will empower you to discuss them with your doctor at your next appointment. Our body doesn't work in isolated silos, so if we take a holistic approach to health problems, they can all be treated at the same time and you can regain your quality of life.

Fibromyalgia

This is a chronic disorder characterized by widespread musculoskeletal pain, which is often described as a burning or aching pain accompanied by fatigue and sleep, memory and mood problems. The cause of fibromyalgia is unclear, but it is thought that repeated nerve stimulation results in changes to the brain and spinal cord, amplifying the painful sensations. Often it will develop following an infection, illness, operation or a period of stress.

What is the link with IBS?

People with IBS are almost twice as likely to suffer from fibromyalgia as non-IBS sufferers. It appears to be most common in people with IBS-M (mixed), followed by IBS-C (see page 19).

Studies have shown that people with fibromyalgia and IBS report worse symptoms of pain, fatigue and morning tiredness compared to those without IBS. At the same time, people with IBS report that their digestive symptoms are worse when they have a flare-up of fibromyalgia. This is consistent with other reports linking the aggravation of digestive symptoms during flare-ups of fibromyalgia.

The gut microbiome is central to both disorders. Studies have shown that a disrupted gut microbiome can exacerbate fibromyalgia symptoms, but can be improved with antibiotic treatment and diet changes.

The gut–brain axis has also emerged as a possible explanation in chronic-pain syndromes.

Chronic fatigue syndrome (CFS)

This is a complicated disorder characterized by extreme fatigue that lasts for at least six months, and which cannot be fully explained by an underlying medical condition. The fatigue becomes worse with physical or mental activity and doesn't improve with rest.

CFS is also known as myalgic encephalomyelitis (ME) or is occasionally abbreviated as ME/CFS. Another recent terminology proposed for this is systemic exertional intolerance disease (SEID).

Symptoms of chronic fatigue syndrome vary from person to person, and the severity of symptoms fluctuates from day to day. Some of the signs and symptoms may include fatigue, memory or concentration problems, sore throat, headaches, enlarged lymph nodes in the neck or armpits, unexplained muscle/joint pain, dizziness that worsens with moving from lying down or sitting to standing, and extreme exhaustion after physical or mental exercise.

The cause of chronic fatigue syndrome is unknown. Many theories exist, however, ranging from viral infections to psychological stressors. You can find out more about chronic fatigue syndrome in another title in the Penguin Life Expert series, called *Living with Chronic Fatigue* by Dr Gerald Coakley and Beverley Knops.

Fatigue is a symptom of many illnesses, infections and psychological disorders. It is always worth making an appointment to see your family doctor if you experience persistent or excessive fatigue. We will probably learn a lot more going forward, because investigation into Long COVID is starting and it bears many similarities to chronic fatigue syndrome.

Migraine headaches

Migraine is a disabling chronic headache, which is defined as recurrent moderate to severe headache attacks lasting from four to seventy-two hours. It can often be accompanied by nausea and/or vomiting. Both migraine and IBS are diagnosed as being more prevalent in young women. One 2021 Polish study found that headache was associated with IBS in 25–50 per cent of subjects.[2]

Migraine is one of the types of headache most commonly associated with IBS. In particular, dysregulation of the gut–brain axis plays a major role. In individuals with IBS, hypersensitivity affects the ENS, which then sends signals to the brain, which in turn makes other parts of the body more sensitive to pain.

> **In pain? Please don't suffer in silence**
> **IBS affects roughly twice as many women as men worldwide, and there are particular challenges for women with IBS. Unfortunately symptoms can worsen around the time of your**

period, so you may well be coping with a double dose of discomfort if you also suffer from pre-menstrual syndrome or primary dysmenorrhoea (period pain). One small UK study of thirty women with IBS found that menstruation was associated with the worsening of abdominal pain and bloating compared with most other phases of the menstrual cycle, and with more frequent bowel habits and a general lower sense of well-being.[3]

I very often sense that some of my female patients downplay the severity of their symptoms for fear of causing a fuss, or believe the discomfort is simply something to put up with. Just recently this gender inequality in medical care has been highlighted, justifiably. In 2021 the UK-based Faculty of Sexual and Reproductive Healthcare reminded healthcare staff of the need to offer women adequate pain relief when having an intrauterine device (IUD) – also known as the coil – fitted, after women spoke out about experiencing pain. Women no longer need to put up with procedural pain and discomfort.

You must not put up with it. Please do raise your concerns. Honesty is the best approach: if you are uncomfortable or in pain, you must speak up, so that you and your doctor can discuss the right management plan for your individual symptoms and circumstances. Chapter 10 has a list of questions to ask your doctor. These have been compiled to help you get the best out of any medical appointment, so that you feel empowered to take treatment into your own hands and have a constructive conversation with your doctor.

The same advice goes for everyone – men, too – if you are due to have any investigations, such as colonoscopy. No exam, test or procedure should make you feel uncomfortable or, worse still, leave you in any pain. No doctor wants to see a patient in pain: talk through options such as sedation or any general pain relief, and don't be dissuaded, if comfort is what you seek.

Temporomandibular disorders (TMDs)

This refers to a group of disorders involving the temporo-mandibular joint (TMJ) – the masticatory or chewing muscles of the jaw. The main symptoms are jaw pain, a clicking sound when the jaw moves and alterations in lower-jaw movements.

Fewer than 10 per cent of people with TMDs seek medical help, and these are mainly women of reproduct-ive age. Studies show that people with IBS are three times more likely to have a TMD risk, irrespective of the type of IBS they have. This increased risk is independent of any specific IBS subtype.

Chronic pelvic pain, interstitial cystitis and dysuria (pain on urination)

Historically, investigations into the causes of chronic pelvic pain have focused on the pelvic organs themselves, to try and find inflammation or infection. More recently, however, studies have indicated that the issue may lie within the central nervous system. Pain in the pelvic region can worsen when you are on your period, urinating, having a bowel movement or after sex.

In addition to chronic pelvic pain, IBS patients are also more likely to suffer from interstitial cystitis, a condition that tends to affect more women than men and which causes long-term pelvic pain, a feeling of pressure and problems in urinating. Patients are also more prone to suffer from other bladder-dysfunction symptoms, such as urge incontinence (when the bladder contracts when it shouldn't, causing an intense need to urinate), pain on urination (dysuria) and wanting to urinate more at night.

This prevalence is quite intriguing, as both the bowel and bladder are served by a similar, but not identical, nerve supply. Colon-only and bladder-only central nerves lie in very close proximity to each other within a part of the spinal cord. This proximity provides potential opportunities for these nerves to communicate with one another. There appears to be an anatomical overlap of peripheral nerves to the bowel and the urinary system. Irritation of the bowel with an inflammatory agent has been shown to lead to an early bladder contraction, triggering the urge to urinate early.

Interestingly, some medications found to help in IBS have been shown to improve bladder dysfunction as well, and further trials are ongoing.

6. The Gut Microbiome Explained

Picture the scene: a large city airport at the start of the summer getaway. Taxis zooming in and out, dropping off and collecting passengers and their luggage. The long, snaking queue at security, the harried passengers dashing through the gate after hearing the final call for their transatlantic flight.

London's Heathrow Airport saw a staggering eighty million passengers pass through its doors in 2018.[1] But the world's busiest transport hubs have nothing on the trillions upon trillions of organisms living and thriving inside our gut, known as the gut microbiome. Over the last fifteen years there has been an explosion of research into this emerging field and the links to IBS, so this book would not be complete without looking at the science behind, and the significance of, the gut microbiome.

The gut microbiome is known to affect our metabolism, immunity, hormones and neural processes. We are also finding new associations between our microbiome and disease processes, from IBS and colorectal cancer, to other conditions such as heart disease and diabetes. Complex names such as Firmicutes and Bacteroidetes, Proteobacteria, Actinobacteria, Prevotella and Ruminococcus are discussed in various health magazines. We know that the composition of the microbiome differs in disease and health, but studies have not yet shown specific abundances in specific disease states. This is still unknown. We are not yet at the point of targeted treatments, as enticing as this may seem.

This chapter takes a deeper look at the gut microbiome and how it affects general health and well-being and, of course, IBS. We will also look at what happens when the microbiome is thrown off-balance, at measures that can help to restore balance and at whether the recent trend for gut-health testing is really worth parting with your money for.

What is the gut microbiome?

The term 'microbiome' refers to the collective mass of one hundred trillion microorganisms of bacteria, viruses, fungi and other life forms that live inside our bodies. To put that into perspective, we have as many microorganisms in our bodies as we do cells living on the surface of our skin, inside our nose and in our gut.

Each area of our body has a distinct microbiome, but the most heavily colonized part of the body is in the GI tract, known as the gut microbiome. The make-up of our gut microbiome varies in different areas of the GI tract: the diversity and density of bacterial species increases as you move down from the mouth, at the top of the GI tract, to the latter parts of the gut.

Why is the gut microbiome so important?

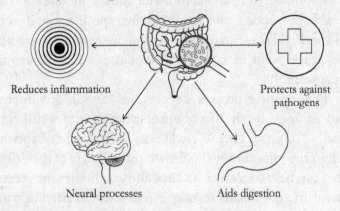

Reduces inflammation

Protects against pathogens

Neural processes

Aids digestion

The role of the gut microbiome

Here are some of the gut microbiome's key functions:

- **Aids digestion**: The bacteria in the microbiome break down dietary fibre, a type of carbohydrate that adds bulk to our foods during the digestive process, making stools easier to pass and preventing constipation (I will be talking about fibre in much more detail in Chapter 8).

- **Reduces inflammation and helps to protect against cancer**: When bacteria in the gut break down fibre, they produce short-chain fatty acids (SCFAs), which are used throughout the body. The three main SCFAs are acetate, butyrate and propionate. **Acetate** helps to keep a healthy pH balance in the gut, and also binds to receptors in

the gut lining to regulate appetite and the storage of fat. **Butyrate** is the main source of energy for the cells in our gut. It has been found to reduce inflammation, and inhibits the production of a protein called HDAC2, which is associated with an increased risk of colorectal cancer.
Propionate also has anti-inflammatory effects throughout the body, and can help to lower cholesterol and blood-sugar levels.

- **Produces vitamins and minerals that we need for survival**: These include **folate**, which helps the body manufacture red and white blood cells in the bone marrow and converts food into energy; **niacin** (vitamin B3), which helps to convert food into energy, can help to lower cholesterol and has anti-inflammatory effects; and **vitamin K**, which helps with blood clotting.

- **Protects against pathogens**: A rich and diverse gut microbiome helps to restrict the presence and growth of disease-causing microorganisms, known as pathogens. These include *Helicobacter pylori*, which can cause stomach ulcers; and harmful strains of *E. coli*, which can cause stomach cramps, vomiting and diarrhoea.

- **Other benefits**: Studies have shown that the gut microbiome also helps to protect the heart, brain and immune system and reduces the risk of Type 2 diabetes.

Symbiosis to dysbiosis: what happens when the gut microbiome is disrupted

The relationship between the gut microbiome and the rest of the body is one of symbiosis, in that they live alongside each other and depend on each other for survival. But when the finely tuned balance of our gut microbiome is disrupted, the composition of the microbiome and its function are affected. This is known as dysbiosis, which can be bad news for our overall health: typically it means a loss of protective microorganisms, excessive growth of potentially harmful organisms and a reduction of overall diversity.[2]

Why does this happen? Our gut microbiome is as individual as we are. And our growing knowledge in this field shows that factors such as our own genes, diet, medications (especially antibiotics) and other environmental factors may lead to a permanent dysbiotic disruption.

Take food, for example: our gut microbiome appears to undergo relatively rapid changes upon exposure to different diets. Western diets are especially high in fat and have high proportions of animal-based foods. Studies have shown that this type of diet can alter the microbiome in just two days.[3]

How does dysbiosis affect IBS?

Research is pointing to the idea that dysbiosis plays a part in the development and severity of symptoms in some people with IBS.

As we covered in Chapter 2, a bout of infection can lead to PI-IBS, while antibiotic use can alter the microbiome. More recently, researchers have been looking at the link between IBS and small-intestinal bacterial overgrowth – a condition where the small intestine becomes colonized with bacteria, causing IBS-like symptoms. Changes in our microbiome composition causing reduced microbial diversity and less SCFA-producing bacteria have been reported in patients with IBS.

Can a change in diet 'heal' my gut microbiome?

A dysbiotic microbiome has been related to several diseases and disorders, including:

- Crohn's disease and ulcerative colitis

- Allergies

- Obesity

- IBS

- Colorectal polyps and colorectal cancers

- Cirrhosis of the liver

- Neurological disorders such as dementia and Parkinson's disease

- Cardiovascular disorders

- Cholesterol gallstones

- Malnutrition

- Kidney disease.[4]

It is yet to be proven whether the microbiome's compositional changes are a cause or a consequence of these diseases. Part of the complexity in this research concerns the vast differences between the microbiomes of apparently healthy people. Combinations of environmental, genetic and lifestyle factors affect our microbes, and the extensive interactions between these microbes and ourselves. The difficulty is that what is a healthy microbiome for one person may not confer health on another. Mind-boggling – really!

A Mediterranean-style diet with plenty of fresh fruits, vegetables and fish, and less red meat, has been shown to have beneficial effects on the gut microbiome. But while it goes without saying that a healthy diet and lifestyle are always recommended for general health, we simply don't know enough about the microbiome to prescribe a definitive formula for what to eat and when, and what to avoid.

In addition, diet is not solely responsible for changes to the gut microbiome. We are coming to understand more and more about the role and effect that our genetic predisposition, early life influences, stress and medication exposures have on the microbiome. However, watch this space: I am optimistic that a greater understanding of our gut microbiome will pave the way for potential approaches to treating and managing IBS alongside existing medication and other symptom-management methods that we use.

What about probiotic supplements?

Probiotics are foods containing live bacteria that are thought to help restore balance in the gut after illness, infection or treatment such as a course of antibiotics. Probiotic sources include live yoghurt, kefir, live apple-cider vinegar and fermented foods such as kombucha, sauerkraut and kimchi.

At the other end of the scale, **prebiotics** are foods that stimulate the growth of 'good' bacteria in the gut, including garlic and onions, ginger and asparagus.

There is a huge market out there, focusing mainly on probiotic foods and supplements available in supermarkets and health-food stores, and many of my own patients with mild IBS do use them. If you are considering taking probiotics, do speak to your family doctor and use them as part of a holistic approach. One option is Symprove, a water-based probiotic. Studies have shown that it is able to survive stomach acids long enough to colonize the gut with good bacteria.[5]

Gut-health testing: why you should avoid it – for now at least

In recent years growing numbers of patients will arrive at their appointments clutching a printout of a report after having had gut-health testing, as in Zara's case overleaf.

Zara, 32

Zara was a self-employed seamstress who came for a
consultation after five long years of significant
abdominal pain. The pain usually started after meals,
but also frequently kept her awake at night. Worryingly,
she lost 12kg (26½ lb) in two years. She explained
that she had seen several naturopaths and alternative
practitioners. She had been diagnosed with a 'leaky gut'
and started on a dairy-free, gluten-free low-FODMAP
diet.

Zara said she saw some improvements, so she
continued with her diet long-term and even started
taking apple-cider vinegar daily, as advised. However, she
began to notice a change in her stools, which became
smaller and harder. She then paid to have expensive stool
tests performed by an independent laboratory. This
resulted in a seventeen-page multicoloured document
proclaiming her to be lacking in several 'good bacteria'
and 'at risk' for several autoimmune conditions.

She was advised to take no fewer than eight different
supplements, all of them (perhaps unsurprisingly)
supplied by the same company, to mitigate her risk. She
followed the advice and purchased the supplements, but
developed skin rashes and worsening pain and bloating
in her abdomen. Zara was afraid to eat anything other
than bone-broth and steamed green vegetables, lest her
symptoms become worse. She was losing weight – and

lost her job because she had taken so much time off sick, due to her symptoms.

During our first appointment it was evident that she was fatigued, appeared depressed and was pale and weak. Her blood tests revealed iron deficiency, vitamin B_{12} and folate deficiency with abnormal liver tests. I asked Zara to resume a normal diet, with small meals six times a day for six weeks. I undertook an upper endoscopy, which showed that her stomach was obviously irritated; and a biopsy from her small intestine revealed that she had coeliac disease. I arranged for a DEXA scan, which looks at bone density, and this showed that she had coeliac disease-related osteoporosis.

It was only after we discussed starting a gluten-free diet, along with the inclusion of all other food groups and an exercise programme, that Zara started to gain weight. It took approximately six months to see her smiling and confident, and no longer scared to socialize. Her business has progressed in leaps and bounds. She will always need to be on a gluten-free diet; however, this has normalized her absorption of all the other vitamins and has enabled her bone strength to improve. Had she continued without a diagnosis despite excluding gluten, she might have suffered the risks of untreated coeliac disease, with nutrient deficiencies, fracture risk and a higher incidence of lymphomas.

Zara's story shows how essential it is that you undertake scientifically proven tests and investigations: expensive does not always equal proven. If you have persistent symptoms it is always worth seeking medical advice. Restricting food groups unnecessarily is not a meaningful way to live and to enjoy long-term quality of life.

Gut-health testing (also known as gut-microbiome testing) involves collecting and sending off a stool sample for analysis, where it is checked for the number and types of bacteria present, to gauge how 'healthy' your gut is. Some tests will look for other markers of gut health, such as calprotectin – a protein that indicates inflammation. Often the testing company includes a free nutritional consultation, with advice to alter your diet or take supplements to improve your health.

Several private companies and websites offer these tests, but this method is not yet used in the UK by the NHS, and with good reason. While I believe that gut-health testing will become a valuable tool for investigating both digestive and systemic conditions in future, the science behind these tests is still in its infancy and we remain in the very early stages of understanding the gut microbiome: we still do not know what the 'optimal' microbiome is and how to manipulate it safely and effectively.

I have looked through several of these reports with my patients, and I have yet to find anything that I would say is useful, either to me as a gastroenterologist or to the patient themselves. I would avoid gut-health testing for the following reasons:

- **Lack of standardization**: Because there is no one standard test, companies can set their own parameters, which means that your results may vary between companies.

- **It is expensive**: Prices vary, but companies may charge upwards of £200 for 'basic' tests, and more still for 'advanced' testing.

- **The results can be misleading**: Some companies create reports that can give unfounded results for the benefits against certain diseases.

- **The tests can cause alarm – or, worse still, offer false reassurance**: Some tests link the presence of certain bacteria to an increased susceptibility of developing a disease. This can be alarming to read, for some patients, and may cause a lot of worry. One stool sample is not enough to tell you if you are at risk of developing cardiovascular disease, diabetes or colon cancer in the future.

- **A 'normal' microbiome has not yet been identified**: A range of companies will give results comparing the bacteria found in your stool with that among the wider population. Because we don't yet know what an optimal microbiome looks like, this isn't particularly useful. Some companies also give percentage values for 'bacterial load', which isn't terribly meaningful.

> To put that into perspective, 1,000 types of bacteria are found in every gram of stool.

In short, there is nothing in these results or reports that you couldn't find out from a proper medical discussion with your family doctor or a gastroenterologist. These tests are merely a single snapshot of the microbes in your stool sample. Currently we cannot say, from levels of stool bacteria, what to eat, or do, or take to alter your symptoms or your risk of disease.

7. Symptom-Based Medication Treatment

Now that we have a deeper understanding of the mechanics of IBS, it is time to move on to the treatments that can help to bring relief of your symptoms. Two questions that I most frequently hear from patients after diagnosis are 'Will I feel like this for the rest of my life?', often quickly followed by 'What are my treatment options?'

While IBS is not life-threatening, it is still a chronic lifelong condition, and unfortunately there is no one pill or powder that will provide an instant cure. The natural cycle of IBS is to have relapsing-remitting (worsening, then improving) symptoms over time, and the focus of any treatment is to manage these symptoms so that you can get on with living the best life possible. The good news is that there is a stable of over-the-counter and prescription treatments out there to try, but it may be that medication isn't always necessary.

If your IBS symptoms are mild to moderate and don't tend to interfere with your everyday life, then you will probably find you can manage your symptoms with the diet and other lifestyle changes that I set out in Chapter 8.

However, if your symptoms are moderate to severe – that is, they are affecting your work, your relationships and family dynamics, and your quality of life – then medication is definitely an option worth exploring. From stool-softeners for constipation, to anti-diarrhoeal agents, in this chapter I will be taking you through all the main over-the-counter and prescription treatments currently available. We will look at how they work, how long they take to show results and whether they have any side-effects.

I will also be looking at newer treatments to emerge in the last decade – and at the so-called 'cures', such as colonic irrigation, that you should definitely avoid.

In addition, I cannot stress how important the relationship you have with your doctor is, at this juncture. Good two-way communication will not only make you feel supported and heard, but also involved in decisions about your treatment every step of the way (for more tips on establishing a good relationship with your doctor, see Chapter 10).

You should be having an open discussion with your doctor about which medicines you should use, whether they are going to be used alongside other treatments and whether they should be used continuously or on a short-term basis. You know your symptoms better than anyone, and your attitude and approach play a huge part in how successful your treatment is. There is a lot to digest in this chapter, but I hope you will be tackling some of these choices with your doctor.

Above all, **you** are the best advocate for your own health. And medical therapies are never a substitute for good lifestyle habits. A prescription medication can never be fully beneficial unless you are well hydrated and nourished. Paying attention to when your body needs the bathroom and giving yourself enough time to have a bowel movement is essential; as well as the need to protect your privacy when going to the bathroom, if this is concerning to you – as many people find this especially difficult at work.

Simple measures alone may make all the difference in some cases. Other avenues, as described in this chapter, are available and have a role in more recalcitrant cases.

I've been diagnosed with IBS – what treatments do I need?

Before I discuss potential treatments, now is a good time to recap on the definition of IBS and the subtypes. As we now know, IBS has a variety of symptoms and subtypes, and treatment should be based on your predominant symptoms and subtype, to give you the best chance of finding relief.

So IBS is recurrent abdominal pain occurring, on average, at least one day per week in the last three months. This will be associated with two or more of the following:

1. Defecation symptoms getting better or worse

2. A change in the frequency of stool

3. A change in the form (appearance) of stool.

IBS is then divided into the following subtypes:

- IBS with predominant constipation (IBS-C)

- IBS with predominant diarrhoea (IBS-D)

- IBS with mixed bowel habits (IBS-M)

- IBS unclassified – this covers those patients who meet the diagnostic criteria for IBS but cannot be accurately categorized into one of the above subtypes.

In the following pages I will be concentrating on medication for IBS-C and IBS-D – that is, the constipation- and diarrhoea-predominant types of IBS. If you have a diagnosis of mixed or unclassified IBS, you will probably need a combined approach of these treatments.

IBS with constipation (IBS-C) treatments

In my experience, many patients with IBS-C will see an improvement in their symptoms from simply increasing their water intake and by upping soluble fibre in their diets. Some also report success from taking powders or supplements made from psyllium, a type of fibre that isn't absorbed by the body, and which adds bulk to stools and relieves constipation (psyllium is also known as ispaghula); it is an easily soluble fibre that is also used for diarrhoea.

However, if these measures fail, the next step is trying some over-the-counter laxatives. Laxatives, a treatment to relieve constipation, are split into two broad groups: osmotic laxatives and stimulant laxatives.

Osmotic laxatives

These work by drawing more water into the bowel from the body. This in turn softens the stool, making it easier to pass. There are two main types of osmotic laxatives: macrogols and lactulose.

- **Macrogol laxatives:** These consist of large molecules that cause the stool to hold and retain water. They are used for constipation as well as the relief of stool impaction (when stools become hard and stuck). They usually come in powder form, to be mixed with a glass of water and taken once daily up to a maximum of twice a day, if needed. They come in various flavours (including a chocolate flavour, if you are so inclined), although many patients say the plain variety is the most palatable.

  Macrogol laxatives are cheap and easily available under brand names such as Movicol, Cosmocol and Laxido. Most patients tolerate macrogol laxatives well because they tend to have fewer side-effects than other osmotic laxatives. However, side-effects can still occur, including abdominal pain, diarrhoea, nausea and flatulence.

  Studies have shown that while this type of laxative will relieve constipation and mean that patients have significantly more spontaneous bowel movements, improved stool consistency and a reduced need to strain, it is less likely to help with abdominal pain or bloating.

Macrogol should not be used for more than one week without medical advice.

- **Lactulose laxatives**: Lactulose is a liquid form of sugar, which is not absorbed by the body, but draws water from the bowel to soften the stool. Taken orally, lactulose works to empty the bowels at a slower rate, with the full laxative effect taking between twelve and forty-eight hours.

  Safe to use in pregnancy, lactulose laxatives are available over the counter, but only in pharmacies rather than supermarkets or other shops. Side-effects may include nausea, vomiting, abdominal pain (usually with higher doses), wind and bloating.

Other types of osmotic laxatives include:

- **Saline laxatives**: These are salt-based, fast-acting laxatives that pull water into the intestines and rapidly empty all the contents of the bowel. They get to work in as little as thirty minutes (and up to three hours). Examples include citrate salts and magnesium preparations such as Milk of Magnesia, sulphate salts and sodium phosphate.

  Saline laxatives are not intended for long-term use as they can lead to dehydration and an imbalance of minerals in the body. If you are advised to use them, make sure you drink plenty of water during their use. Saline laxatives are not suitable for people with kidney disease or those taking medication to lower their sodium levels.

- **Glycerine suppositories**: This treatment has an osmotic effect in drawing water, and glycerine also acts as a mild stimulant, causing the bowel muscles to contract and making it easier for the body to pass the stool. The suppositories will usually result in a bowel movement within fifteen minutes to an hour after insertion, so you may find it better to use them first thing in the morning when the natural urge to empty your bowels is at its strongest. Alternatively the suppositories can work overnight, so you may want to try using them before bed.

  You might be nervous about using a suppository, but patients tend to find glycerine suppositories straightforward to use, without any major side-effects. However, possible side-effects include some burning or irritation around the anus after insertion, abdominal pain and cramps.

Over-the-counter laxatives: five top tips for success

1. If you have ongoing chronic constipation, it is best to seek the help of a medical professional before self-treating with over-the-counter laxatives.
2. Read the enclosed instruction leaflet carefully and, if in doubt, ask a pharmacist for advice.
3. Do not be tempted to exceed the stated dose.
4. Keep hydrated: with all laxatives it is important to drink at least 1.5l (2½ pt) of

water daily, plus an additional 100ml (3½ fl. oz) glass with every laxative dose taken, to prevent dehydration.

5. Never use an over-the-counter laxative for more than a week, unless advised to do so by a healthcare professional: once medically advised, prolonged laxative use may be appropriate under some circumstances. Laxative abuse, however, describes the chronic overuse of laxatives for purposes other than relieving constipation. This may be due to an eating disorder, a factitious disorder or Munchausen's syndrome, whereby patients seek out unnecessary investigations.

Long-term laxative abuse can lead to serious dysfunction of bowel motility, such as cathartic colon (also known as lazy or laxative gut). Cathartic colon describes the anatomical and physiological changes in the colon that occur with the long-term use of stimulant laxatives. This causes symptoms of abdominal pain, bloating, a sensation of fullness and incomplete bowel evacuation. There are also irreversible and severely damaging effects of laxative abuse, such as kidney failure, liver damage and bowel nerve damage. Therefore it is important to use laxatives only in moderation and under the supervision of a doctor or healthcare provider.

Stimulant laxatives

Stimulant laxatives are used for the fast relief of constipation. They work by increasing peristalsis, the normal muscular contractions of the digestive tract. This means that stool moves faster, and the amount of liquid is increased.

These laxatives are widely available over the counter, and I find that a lot of patients will have already tried them before coming to see me. However, I would urge caution: stimulant laxatives should only be used under the recommendation of a pharmacist or healthcare professional. In addition to side-effects such as nausea, long-term use can lead the body to become dependent on them for a bowel movement.

- **Senna**: Senna is the pod or leaf of the plant *Senna alexandrina* and is commonly used in laxatives. Senna contains chemicals called sennosides, which stimulate the lining of the bowel and cause a laxative effect.

  Senna tablets are probably the most common over-the-counter laxative available in supermarkets and pharmacies. In fact many shops stock their own brand. Most brands will contain 7.5mg of Sennoside B, the active ingredient, while 'max-strength' formulations contain twice this dose. Senna is also found in various teas and liquid formulations.

  It can be safely used in children as well as adults, but is not recommended for use during pregnancy.

- **Bisacodyl:** Commonly known in the UK as the brand Dulcolax, bisacodyl is another stimulant laxative found in many supermarket 'constipation relief' formulations. Bisacodyl comes in both tablet and suppository form. The usual dose is 5–10mg in tablet form, usually taken at night before bed, and a 10mg suppository used first thing in the morning.

Other treatments for IBS-C

- **Stool softeners:** These act to increase the water and fat content of the stool, making it softer and easier to pass. This also greatly reduces or eliminates the need to strain. In addition to IBS, stool softeners may be recommended after childbirth or surgery, or during a bout of haemorrhoids. The main stool softener is docusate sodium (known by the brand name Colace in the US and Dulcoease in the UK) and it comes in liquid or capsule form. Stool softeners are mild in nature, but may cause abdominal cramps. Some patients report developing a mild tolerance to stool softeners and may require higher doses over time.

- **Enemas:** An enema involves the rectal insertion of liquid, which could be water or a salt solution, which acts as a mechanical and osmotic stimulant. It can be used to relieve severe constipation and empty the bowel prior to surgery.

There are prepared enemas available at most pharmacies. Once the liquid is inserted, it is necessary to try to hold this in place for a few minutes until there is an intense urge to open your bowels. Enemas may cause uncomfortable bloating and cramping; however, they usually work well to eliminate the contents of the bowel in a short period of time.

Why you should avoid colonic irrigation

A colonic irrigation, or colon cleansing, involves 'flushing' out the colon with large amounts of water (which is sometimes mixed with herbs or even coffee) via a tube inserted into the rectum. My advice? Save your money.

Colonic irrigations are popular, especially amongst alternative-medicine practitioners, but are widely viewed with distrust by the conventional medical community. A quick internet search will bring up numerous advertisements and websites recommending colonic irrigation to improve bowel motility and reduce constipation. Yet there is a complete lack of medical evidence for these claims.

Other perceived benefits of colonic irrigation are that it helps to 'detoxify' the body, aids weight loss and digestion and improves energy – and even reduces the risk of cancer. Again there is no evidence to back up these claims, and no physician or healthcare professional will recommend this practice.

In addition, the risks of colonic irrigation include:

- Dehydration
- Perforation of the rectum or bowel from the equipment being used
- Disruption to the balance of electrolytes, such as calcium, potassium and magnesium: all essential minerals that maintain fluid balance in the body and regulate functions, including blood pressure and muscle contractions. This can be particularly dangerous if you have heart or kidney disease.
- Infection: In the late 1970s and early 1980s an outbreak of amoebiasis – a disease where the intestines become infected with the single-cell parasite *Entamoeba histolytica* – at an American clinic offering colonic irrigation resulted in seven deaths.[1] The case subsequently led to the adoption of single-use/disposable devices in colonic irrigation.

I appreciate that constipation can be miserable, but I would urge you not to go down the route of colonic irrigation. Please consult a doctor first. It may be that there is a medical treatment you haven't yet explored, or that you need to give your current treatment more time to work.

- **Lubricant laxatives:** These are oily laxatives, using ingredients such as paraffin oil to coat the colon and stool in a waterproof film. This enables it to become soft and easier to pass, usually within six to eight hours. Lubricant laxatives are used less frequently, as they have been shown to have limited therapeutic value. Some have been shown to cause vitamin A, D, E and K deficiencies, and they may also interfere with the absorption of other medications. Small amounts of them may also cause lung damage, such as lipoid pneumonia, a rare but serious disease where fat or oil get into the lungs.

Prescription medication for IBS-C

Many new medications have emerged in the last couple of decades for the treatment of IBS.

Gut-targeted pharmacotherapy

Gut-targeted medicines target colonic tissue and are used in IBS-C, often with extremely good effect.

Guanylate cyclase agonists are licensed for the treatment of moderate to severe IBS-C associated with constipation. They work by increasing bowel secretions and movement so that stools are easier to pass, as well as helping to ease abdominal pain. They are currently available on prescription in the UK as Linaclotide, which is taken as a 290mcg capsule once daily; it is also known as Constella. In the US and Mexico it is named Linzess and is available in 72mcg, 145mcg and 290mcg doses.

This class of medication is proven to be effective, safe and well tolerated. Studies show that patients taking Linaclotide demonstrated significant improvement in abdominal pain/discomfort, bloating, straining and stool consistency, as well as the number of spontaneous bowel movements per week, when compared to a placebo. The main side-effect – perhaps to be expected – is diarrhoea, which only required 6 per cent of patients to discontinue its use.[2]

5-hydroxytryptamine (serotonin) 4 receptor agonists

Most of us are aware of the importance of the hormone serotonin in regulating our mood and our sense of happiness. But 90 per cent of serotonin produced by our body is actually found in our stomach and intestines. Serotonin (5-HT) is a vital neurotransmitter, or chemical messenger, that controls gut motor and sensory function.

Recent advances in the treatment of IBS include therapies that help to regulate serotonin levels and activity. In IBS-C the aim is to stimulate serotonin receptors in the gut, particularly the serotonin type-4 receptor (known as 5-HT4). This helps to promote peristalsis and accelerate the movement of stools through the gut.[3]

One such medication is Prucalopride, which not only stimulates serotonin receptors, but does not tend to have the same side-effects as laxatives.[4] Available in the UK and the US (where it is known as Motegrity), Prucalopride is recommended as an option for chronic constipation only in women (because clinical trials didn't have enough males taking part to prove its effectiveness). It can be used only when treatment with at least two laxatives from different classes, at the highest tolerated recommended doses for at least six months, has failed to provide adequate relief.

A partial 5-HT4 agonist (Tegaserod) was approved for use in the United States in 2002 in tablet form at 2mg or 6mg, under the brand name Zelnorm. The typically recommended dose was 2–6mg twice daily. Unfortunately, Tegaserod was withdrawn in 2007 because of adverse cardiovascular side-effects. It is still used, but only on an emergency basis and with prior authorization from the US Food and Drug Administration (FDA), although these limitations are being contested.

Prucalopride has been safely used for years and has not been associated with similar problems.

Lubiprostone (Amitiza)

This is a type of drug called a chloride-channel activator, which increases the secretion of fluid into the bowel, making stools softer and easier to pass. Amitiza capsules were discontinued for use in the UK in 2019, and there is currently no other medication containing lubiprostone available. However, Amitiza is still available on prescription in other countries, including the US.

Other medications

There are other new medications currently in clinical trials, which may be approved for treatment of IBS-C in the UK in the future. Some of them are already available in other countries, including tenapanor, which was approved for use in the US in 2019. Known under the brand name Ibsrela, tenapanor is a type of drug called a sodium/hydrogen exchanger 3 (NHE3) inhibitor. These drugs reduce absorption of sodium from the small intestine and colon, and increase secretion of fluid into the bowel, so that stools are softer and easier to pass. Two studies have also found that tenapanor helps to ease abdominal pain.

IBS with diarrhoea (IBS-D) treatments

As with the treatment of IBS-C, there are a number of over-the-counter and prescription treatments available. They include anti-diarrhoeal agents and bile-acid sequestrants.

Anti-diarrhoeal agents

These medications work by altering the muscular activity of the intestine, thereby prolonging the time it takes for contents to pass through. *Note*: They are generally not helpful long-term for those with IBS-M, and you should avoid taking them altogether if you have IBS-C.

- **Loperamide (also known as Imodium or Imodium A-D):** This is a synthetic agent that inhibits peristalsis. It is also used for faecal incontinence as it helps tighten the anal sphincter. Several trials involving patients with IBS-D have found loperamide is effective in reducing stool frequency and improving stool consistency, but it appears to have no effect on symptoms of abdominal discomfort or bloating.

  Loperamide should only be used in limited doses, and solely on an as-needed basis. It should not be taken for longer than one week without medical advice.

- **Opioid agents, including Lomotil:** You may well have used opioids in the past to relieve pain or after a surgical procedure, but opioids also play a role in slowing gut transit in IBS-D. Lomotil is a prescription-only medication that contains a combination of an opioid called diphenoxylate, plus atropine. Diphenoxylate is similar to opioid pain relievers, but in this case works to slow down the gut. Atropine is a type of medicine called an anticholinergic, which blocks receptors on the surface of muscle cells in the intestine that cause the muscles to contract. Blocking these cell receptors helps to relax the muscles of the intestinal wall and slows down gut movement.

  Another medication that can be prescribed to control diarrhoea is codeine phosphate.

As with other opioid medications, these
treatments carry the risk of addiction, and can
impair performance of tasks such as driving.
Therefore they should be used cautiously and
only under medical advice.

Bile-acid sequestrants

To recap, bile acids are components in our bile made in
the liver, stored in the gall bladder and released into the
small intestine when food is eaten. They help to break
down and absorb fats and vitamins in our food, as well as
remove waste products.

Almost all (about 97 per cent) of our bile acids are
absorbed in the last part of the small intestine (known as
the ileum) and are returned to the liver. But when this
cycle is disturbed, it is called bile-acid malabsorption
(BAM) or bile-acid diarrhoea. BAM affects about one in
every 100 people, although this rises to about one in three
for those with IBS-D.

A diagnostic test to measure the bile-acid reabsorption,
called a SeHCAT (selenium homocholic acid taurine)
scan (see page 54), should be performed before trying
these medications. *Note*: The SeHCAT test is not available in the US, but blood tests are.

Bile-acid sequestrants work by binding to the bile acid
in the small intestine, so they stop the acid irritating the
large intestine. By effectively mopping up the bile acid,
this leads to a firmer stool.[5] Bile-acid sequestrant medications are prescription-only and include cholestyramine

(Questran), colestipol or colesevelam. Cholestyramine comes in powder sachets to be mixed with liquid and is the most commonly used bile-acid sequestrant in the UK. However, some people find it unpalatable and prefer colesevelam, which is available as a tablet.

> **Tip:** If you suffer from bile-acid diarrhoea, it is a good idea to keep to a low-fat diet, as your body has a hard time digesting fat and this can exacerbate your diarrhoea.

Targeted pharmacotherapy

As with IBS-C, in recent years there have been new treatment options for IBS-D, and the key types are listed below. They are all very useful, safe treatments, if prescribed appropriately with adequate follow-up from a doctor.

- **Eluxadoline:** This works by binding to opioid receptors to slow down the movement of the contents of the gut. Although no longer available in the UK or the European Union, it is available in other countries, such as the US and Canada. It isn't recommended for people with liver damage, heavy alcohol use or those who have had their gall bladder removed.

- **Serotonin antagonists:** In IBS-C the aim is to stimulate serotonin receptors in the gut. But the opposite is true when trying to manage diarrhoea-predominant IBS. Drugs known as

5-hydroxytryptamine (serotonin) 3 receptor antagonists work by actively blocking serotonin receptors to reduce motility and ease abdominal pain.

Available on prescription in the US under the brand name Alosetron, this is used to treat severe diarrhoea-predominant IBS in females whose symptoms have lasted for six months and who have failed to respond to all other treatments. Both Alosetron and another serotonin antagonist, Cilansetron, have a proven global improvement in IBS symptoms, with relief of abdominal pain and discomfort.[6]

However, there were some serious side-effects and complications in the initial use of this medication, and as a result Alosetron is now prescribed at a lower starting dose than was previously approved in the US. This is only available under restricted conditions, and by doctors enrolled in the Alosetron prescribing programme.

Stefania, 24

Young investment banker Stefania was flying high professionally, but when it came to her health, she was at a low ebb. She came to see me complaining of sharp abdominal pain, particularly after eating, along with nausea. The symptoms had been ongoing for about a year and were adding to the pressure of her already highly stressful job.

Before coming to see me, Stefania had drastically altered her diet to exclude gluten and dairy. As a result, she had lost 6kg (13¼ lb) in weight. The pain and symptoms were severely hampering her quality of life. Stefania admitted that she was scared to go out and socialize because she was experiencing soft stools up to three times a day, and she was unable to sleep at night because of the pain. The only thing that seemed to help was exercise.

I went through Stefania's medical history and she had a family history of depression through her mother and her sister, who had an underactive thyroid. She became very tearful during our consultation – a combination, she said, of discussing her symptoms in the open and because she felt the two previous doctors she had seen about her symptoms hadn't taken her seriously. Sadly, this is something I hear all too often from my patients with IBS.

I arranged further investigations, including an endoscopy and a colonoscopy, which were normal. Bloods revealed low vitamin D, but did not show signs of coeliac disease or issues with thyroid function.

Stefania was resistant to the idea, but I advised her to stop the exclusion diet she had been following and revert to a normal, balanced diet, but eating little and often. During our discussions she would explain how her symptoms would improve at the weekend, only to worsen again on a Sunday night. We discussed ways of easing work-related stress and alternating her work patterns. After much discussion, she agreed to trialling very low-dose antidepressants, which are often used for IBS. I reassured her that these were not addictive and were not a lifelong treatment, but would take one to two months to see a benefit.

We had a follow-up every month and gradually, by month four, Stefania was sleeping slightly better and was able to eat more foods. We mutually agreed that she would continue her medications, which she tolerated well.

A year on from our first appointment, Stefania was happier, sleeping well and had regained the weight she had lost on her exclusion diet. It took the first six months to gain her confidence in our medical management plan, while the following six months enabled her to regain her appetite for socializing, free from worry about her symptoms. By now Stefania was thriving and was ready to come off her medications, had a healthier relationship with food, and was able to see how excluding foods without proper guidance had only served to increase her anxieties.

Antibiotics

Rifaximin is an oral non-absorbable antibiotic used for the treatment of patients with IBS-D. This is based on the theory that at least a portion of patients with IBS-D have an abnormal microbiome. Rifaximin has been proven in multiple clinical trials to be a safe and effective treatment choice for patients with IBS-D symptoms. It is also known as Xifaxan (US) and Zaxine (Canada). In the UK it is only licensed for use in traveller's diarrhoea, so when prescribed as a treatment for small-intestine bacterial overgrowth (SIBO), rifaximin can only be accessed via private prescription, which can be quite costly.

Treatments for abdominal pain and bloating

Abdominal pain and bloating are seen in patients with all types of IBS. The first line treatment for abdominal pain comprises **antispasmodics** – drugs that relax the muscles of the gut. For patients with abdominal pain due to IBS, we use antispasmodics on an as-needed basis. In patients with IBS-C, antispasmodics may be utilized only if abdominal pain persists despite adequate treatment of the constipation.

If you find you have persistent abdominal pain despite antispasmodics, it is worth discussing with your doctor trying out 'pain modifiers', which are low-dose **antidepressants** used to reduce the sensitivity of the gut nerves.

What are antispasmodics?

Antispasmodics block the transmission of nerve impulses within the gut, relaxing the smooth muscle of the intestines and reducing gut motility. Relaxing the tense muscles relieves spasms of the smooth muscle and the resultant abdominal pain. What makes this medication particularly beneficial is that it provides relief by eliminating the cause, rather than masking the pain.

The main antispasmodic drug is Hyoscine butylbromide, usually known by the brand name Buscopan, which has been used for many decades and is a tried-and-tested, safe and reliable medication that is readily available over the counter. Other examples are Mebeverine hydrochloride and Alverine citrate. Peppermint oil can also help relieve spasms (see Chapter 9 for more information).[7]

Antidepressants

I find that many patients are initially reluctant even to discuss antidepressants: they come to see me with a physical problem, and as soon as I mention antidepressants, some patients feel uncomfortable because they only associate this treatment with mental health. Understandably, some concerns centre around habituation, side-effects, daytime drowsiness and interactions with other medications – nothing that can't be fully explained. However, there is more to antidepressants than their use in helping to treat clinical depression.

I always stress to my patients, when I bring antidepressants into the conversation, that we are not talking about treating depression, but rather that antidepressants are a very useful treatment to have in our armoury, due to their pain-relieving, or analgesic, effects.[8] Antidepressants work by targeting the pain pathways found in the gut. I tend to refer to antidepressants as 'pain modifiers' in my conversations with patients, to make the distinction between their use for pain relief and their general use for mental health and mood.

When I prescribe pain modifiers for abdominal pain in IBS, I always start at a very low dose. This is because there is a slow onset of action for these medications, so it is worth assessing the response at least four to six weeks in, to see if the dose needs adjusting.

There are two particular types of 'pain modifier' that can be beneficial for people with IBS-related abdominal pain:

1. **Tricyclic antidepressants (TCAs)**: These are also known as neuromodulators, and are also used to relieve painful conditions such as fibromyalgia, chronic headaches and diabetic neuropathy.[9] In addition, TCAs slow gut transit, so they are useful for diarrhoea-predominant IBS. It might be stating the obvious, but they should be used with caution if you suffer from constipation. Examples include amitriptyline, nortriptyline, imipramine and desipramine. If one is not tolerated, it is worth trying another.

2. **Selective serotonin reuptake inhibitors (SSRIs) and serotonin-norepinephrine reuptake inhibitors (SNRIs)**: These have less proven data in studies and there have been somewhat inconsistent results over the years,

perhaps in part due to study design. They are, however, used in general for the treatment of IBS in patients in whom depression is a co-factor.[10]

Antibiotics

There is one specific example of use of an antibiotic in patients with moderate to severe IBS especially with abdominal bloating, without constipation, who have failed other therapies, such as low-FODMAP diets, antispasmodics and TCAs. This is a two-week treatment with rifaximin. Studies showed that rifaximin was more effective than a placebo for global IBS symptom improvement, as well as more likely to decrease bloating compared with a placebo.[11] In general, no other antibiotics are used in IBS, although some practitioners will prescribe Neomycin for SIBO treatment as it is cheaper than rifaximin. The non-absorbable nature of rifaximin gives it its excellent safety profile and it is by far the preferred treatment option.

Patients who received rifaximin reported continued relief of symptoms during follow-up, and this treatment can be repeated up to three times.[12]

8. Dietary and Psychological Treatments

We know that IBS is far from being a one-size-fits-all diagnosis. And there is much more to the management of IBS than over-the-counter and prescription medication. It starts with choosing the right doctor for discussion. The doctor–patient relationship can itself be therapeutic, because having greater confidence in your diagnosis and treatment will go a long way towards relieving symptoms.

IBS demands a holistic approach that includes treatment suited to your symptoms, but also looking at how your diet and lifestyle feed into your condition. Food can be a minefield when it comes to IBS: more than four out of five people with IBS report food-related symptoms, especially in relation to certain types of carbohydrates and fats.[1]

Eating should be something to be savoured and enjoyed with others. Do you find yourself skipping meals in company, or does eating leave you feeling sluggish or in pain? If that sounds familiar, then read on. From upping your soluble-fibre intake to establishing a regular eating pattern, in this chapter we will be looking at some straightforward dietary changes that you can start implementing today.

We'll also be looking at the FODMAP diet – a plan that, under the care of a dietician, can pinpoint hard-to-digest foods that may be the source of much discomfort.

Of course a holistic approach to IBS doesn't end with a balanced diet. Exercise is also crucial, so I have included advice on how movement can help ease symptoms such as wind and constipation, plus the best exercises to try.

Finally, we'll also be looking at the impact of mental health on IBS, and how some simple strategies can empower you to better cope with your symptoms.

An IBS-friendly diet

We are what we eat, as the old adage goes. And when it comes to IBS, your diet is crucial: eating the right things for your condition can have an impact on your stool consistency and on symptoms such as wind and bloating. Filling up on the wrong foods, though, can exacerbate your symptoms, leaving you in pain, discomfort and, very likely, fed up. There are, however, pitfalls to avoid in making your diet very restrictive.

As we have seen, more than 80 per cent of people with IBS report food-related symptoms.[2] This is not, however, due to the food itself. Rather it is due to the act of eating and the digestive process, which is kick-started the moment you take a bite of food. Remember, your food is not digested immediately, and meal-related symptoms are not necessarily down to the food groups themselves.

Making sensible and healthy food choices – and really thinking about what, how and when you eat – will give you greater control over your symptoms and should in turn improve your quality of life.

Why allergy tests are unnecessary

It is completely natural that when diagnosed with a health condition like IBS, people look for the root cause so that they can try and fix it. But sometimes that desire to find a solution leads people to look for a problem that isn't necessarily there.

A lot of my patients will ask me if they need tests to rule out whether their symptoms are caused by an allergy. But while skin-prick or blood tests are routinely used by allergists in diagnosing food allergies, they aren't required in the diagnosis and management of IBS. Put simply, a food allergy does not cause IBS; it is a specific immune response to a substance that your body perceives as a threat, such as peanuts, shellfish, milk or eggs.

An allergic reaction is usually instant, with telltale red-flag signs such as itching inside the mouth and throat, hives and swelling of the face. And in some cases a food allergy can be life-threatening. More common are food intolerances, which are harder to diagnose (see below). In fact only 1 per cent of adults will experience a true food allergy. If you have any red-flag symptoms, as described above, do seek medical advice.

So how can diet affect IBS?

The best diet for your microbiome is a varied, colourful, all-inclusive diet with fruits and vegetables of all shapes and sizes – think bitter melon/karela, a staple in Asian dishes, mooli (a large, mild radish also known as daikon), purple asparagus and dark, leafy cavolo nero.

A largely plant-based diet is excellent for providing prebiotics for your gut microbes, which will then thrive and keep diseases at bay. If you restrict your diet, the microbiome is likely to suffer, diminish in its diversity and start to become imbalanced, which may in turn lead to IBS-type symptoms.

What about food-intolerance testing?

As opposed to food allergies, as described above, food intolerance is never life-threatening. It is not triggered by our immune system. Symptoms often occur gradually, a few hours after eating the culprit food, and usually if it is taken in larger quantities. Many different foods can cause intolerances.

There are numerous companies that offer food-intolerance tests commercially. They often produce colourful, expensive and very detailed reports, which offer little scientifically proven information, let alone a true diagnosis. I may be sounding like a broken record here, but my advice is to save your money – and the same goes for hair-analysis or IgG (immunoglobulin G) blood-testing.

If you are concerned about intolerances, it is best to keep a food diary, see what happens when you avoid a specific food group and then reintroduce it again. You should then discuss these results with your family doctor, if problems persist.

Alternative and traditional allergy tests

Traditional allergy tests for true food allergies are scientifically proven, evidence-based and are performed by registered health professionals. They include:

1. **Skin prick tests**: If positive, these tests result in a small swollen lump known as a 'wheal', highlighting an IgE (immunoglobulin E)-mediated food allergy. A clinical history is taken to analyse the full picture.

2. **Blood tests**: Radioallergosorbent tests (RAST) measure levels of IgE antibodies to the common suspected food triggers in the blood. Again, a clinical history is important to corroborate the diagnosis.

3. **Food challenges**: These involve giving the foods to which you have a suspected allergy by mouth, in small amounts. This is then increased while the symptoms are observed. However, these tests must only be performed under

medical supervision where resuscitation equipment is available.

4. **Food exclusion and reintroduction**: This can be very time consuming and is best performed under the supervision of a registered dietician, to ensure a well-balanced nutritional intake during the test period.

Establish a regular eating pattern

An important part of any consultation is discussing diet and eating habits, and it is common for patients to tell me how they regularly miss breakfast, leave long gaps between meals or eat big meals very late at night. And, like our case study of Rachel in Chapter 2, others admit to skipping meals to avoid embarrassing symptoms while at work or when out with friends.

Keep a food diary for a few days to see if any unhelpful patterns emerge. Ask yourself: how often do you skip breakfast, or wolf down your lunch? How does it make you feel afterwards? Consistency is key to managing your symptoms, and that means regular meals – breakfast, lunch, dinner, and snacks where needed. Skipping meals will leave you hungry, irritable and liable to make unwise food choices when you finally sit down to eat.

We all lead busy lives, but try to take time to sit down, chew and enjoy your food. Chewing helps to break down food into more manageable pieces to digest, and signals to your brain that the digestion process is about to begin.

One Iranian study found that insufficient chewing, having fewer teeth and eating spicy foods all increase the likelihood of developing IBS.[3]

Watch your caffeine intake

Caffeine is a stimulant that increases gut motility and can lead to loose stools and/or diarrhoea. It also increases the levels of the stress hormone cortisone, so it could be a factor if stress exacerbates your IBS symptoms.

Current advice is to avoid having more than three cups of tea or coffee a day, but it is worth bearing in mind that different drinks contain varying amounts of caffeine. A 200ml (7 fl. oz) cup of strong instant coffee contains about 90mg of caffeine, a cup of filter coffee contains 140mg, while a cup of medium-strength tea has about 40mg.[4]

Also remember that caffeine is present in other foods, including chocolate – about 33mg in 50g (1¾ oz) of dark chocolate, and 12mg in milk chocolate. Check the ingredients on your over-the-counter medicines, too: some painkillers containing paracetamol and ibuprofen may have caffeine added to improve their efficacy. A 2014 review found that adding 100mg of caffeine to a standard dose of common painkillers improved pain relief by a small but significant 5–10 per cent.[5]

. . . and ditch the fizzy drinks in favour of water

Carbonated drinks, including sparkling water, can induce gas and bloating in your already-sensitized gut. Not only are fizzy drinks likely to include caffeine, but diet versions commonly include sorbitol, an artificial sweetener also found in sugar-free sweets (such as chewing gum) and some slimming products. Sorbitol is poorly absorbed by the gut and can have a laxative effect, so it is best avoided if you suffer from diarrhoea.

Since human beings comprise 90 per cent water, having enough fluid is essential for a well-functioning gut. Water aids the passage of food through the GI tract and helps to prevent dehydration in people with diarrhoea. You should be aiming for eight cups of fluid a day (about 1.5–2l/2½–3½ pt). Water is best, or other non-caffeinated drinks – for example, herbal teas. If you find that water causes bloating, try sipping it throughout the day rather than draining a whole glass in one go.

Watch your alcohol intake, too: alcohol can irritate the gut, prevent absorption of nutrients from food, is dehydrating and can lead to looser stools or diarrhoea. Current guidelines say that men and women should not drink more than fourteen units a week on a regular basis. To put this into perspective, fourteen units equal about 3½l (6 pt) of average-strength beer or ten small glasses of wine.[6]

Manage your fibre intake

We all need fibre in our diets, and eating the right amount and type is essential for people with IBS. Too much of one type and you risk exacerbating symptoms such as diarrhoea and wind, while too little can lead to constipation and discomfort.

Fibre is a type of carbohydrate and is the part of fruits, vegetables and grains that cannot be digested. It is this indigestibility that makes fibre a key issue in both normal functioning of the GI tract and in functional disorders like IBS. It helps digestion by adding bulk to our foods, prevents constipation, helps us feel fuller and encourages the growth of good bacteria in the gut. Wider health benefits include a link to a lower risk of bowel cancer, cardiovascular disease and Type 2 diabetes.

Perhaps most importantly, there are two types of fibre:

- **Soluble fibre**: This dissolves in water to make a gel-like substance that slows digestion and helps form softer, bulkier stools that are easier to pass. This type of fibre can be helpful if you suffer from constipation.

- **Insoluble fibre**: This does not dissolve in water, is tougher and more fibrous. It moves more quickly through the GI tract, helping other foods and liquids to pass speedily along with it.

> **How much fibre do I need, and how do I get it?**
> Current UK guidelines recommend that adults should be eating about 30g (1 oz) of dietary fibre as part of a healthy diet: about 25–30g for women and 30–35g for men. As a guide, two slices of wholemeal bread contain about 5g of fibre.
>
> While symptoms vary from person to person, the general rule is to avoid insoluble fibre if you

have IBS. Soluble fibre is easier to tolerate and should be optimized in people with IBS. The important thing is to adjust your intake gradually over time and assess what works for you.

Good sources of soluble fibre include oat bran, barley, nuts, seeds, legumes and some fruits and vegetables with the skins removed. Sources of insoluble fibre include wholegrains such as wholewheat pasta, bulgur wheat and brown rice.

If you are increasing the amount of fibre in your diet, slow and steady is the way to go. Introducing a large amount in a short space of time can lead to bloating and wind. Guidelines suggest starting at around 3–4g a day and building up gradually to avoid bloating.[7] If you do suffer from wind or bloating, it may help to eat oats (for example, an oat-based breakfast cereal or porridge) and linseeds (up to one tablespoon a day).

Cook from fresh, where possible

Ready meals may be convenient, but they can be a mine-field for people with IBS. As a rule, they are higher in sugar, salt and fat, and low in fibre. A 2018 study showed that adults with diets high in ultra-processed foods and beverages were at higher risk of developing IBS.[8] Cooking your own meals from scratch gives you greater control over the ingredients – and over your symptoms, as a result. If time is short, try batch-cooking your meals.

Keep your gut in mint condition

Mint (*Mentha piperita*) has been used for centuries for ailments including headaches, colds and to freshen breath. But there is now compelling evidence that peppermint oil – an essential oil derived from the peppermint plant – can help to ease symptoms of IBS.

It is thought that peppermint has an antispasmodic, or relaxing, effect on the smooth muscle in the gut, which is responsible for the movement of food by peristalsis. There are other benefits from peppermint, such as reducing visceral sensitivity, and direct antimicrobial and anti-inflammatory effects. Furthermore, studies have found that peppermint oil exerts effects throughout the gut, including on the oesophagus, stomach, small bowel, gall bladder and colon.[9] The only caveat is to use peppermint cautiously if you suffer from heartburn.

Studies have also shown that enteric-coated capsules, which allow peppermint oil to pass through the stomach so that it dissolves in the intestines, may help to relieve abdominal pain, gas and bloating. One review of nine studies of 726 people found that 69 per cent of patients who took peppermint-oil capsules had improved symptoms, compared to 31 per cent of those who received a placebo.[10]

Peppermint-oil capsules are available over the counter, but as with any medicine, do discuss them with a health professional before taking them. The capsules should not be broken or chewed, because peppermint oil may irritate the mouth or oesophagus, while non-enteric peppermint-oil capsules may cause or exacerbate heartburn.

As someone who is partial to a cup of peppermint tea, I also recommend drinking it liberally for the twenty-four hours after an endoscopic procedure to reduce the wind-cramps that may occur. Peppermint tea is an excellent smooth-muscle relaxer through its effects on blocking the gut-calcium channels.

The FODMAP diet: what you need to know

If you have tried the above diet principles without success, the next step could be speaking to your doctor about the FODMAP diet. First devised by scientists at Monash University in Melbourne, Australia, the FODMAP diet is now recommended worldwide as an effective diet for managing IBS symptoms.

FODMAP stands for fermentable oligosaccharides, disaccharides, monosaccharides and polyols. These are short-chain carbohydrates, or sugars, that are found in a variety of foods we eat, including wheat, some fruit and vegetables, pulses, artificial sweeteners and some processed foods.

The issue with FODMAPs is that our bodies have a hard time digesting them. FODMAPs are poorly absorbed in the small intestine and pass into the large intestine, where they are fermented by bacteria. This produces gas that can stretch the already-sensitive bowel, leading to bloating, wind and discomfort or pain. FODMAPs can also draw water into the colon, causing diarrhoea.

Simply put, the FODMAP diet is a personalized diet that avoids the specific FODMAPs that can trigger your symptoms, replacing them with alternatives that are easier to digest. Studies show that the FODMAP diet can have up to a 70 per cent success rate in reducing IBS symptoms.

Despite these accolades for the low-FODMAP diet, studies have shown that an IBS diet has similar effects and is not as restrictive. It can also be undertaken without dietetic advice. An IBS diet essentially means what I have outlined above: that is, small frequent meals, not missing meals and keeping your caffeine intake to three cups per day. I ask patients to follow the IBS diet initially, and to reserve the FODMAP diet for recalcitrant symptoms. This is mostly because a very restricted diet is not beneficial for our microbiome, and should definitely not be prolonged after eight weeks, due to the risk of malnutrition. It is also a daunting, difficult diet to follow, with the exclusion of some wonderful fruits and vegetables;

furthermore, it needs ongoing dietetic support to avoid the risk of malnutrition.

What foods are high in FODMAPs?

This is not a definitive list, but gives you an idea of the types of foods that are high in FODMAPs. Ingredients in processed food and drink can vary from country to country, so this is another reason why you should only undertake the FODMAP diet under the direction of a dietician.

- **Fruit**: Dried fruit, apples, peaches, pears, plums, fruit juice

- **Vegetables**: Artichoke, asparagus, broccoli, cauliflower, garlic, leeks, onion

- **Dairy and alternatives**: Cow's milk, yoghurt, soy milk (made with whole soya beans), condensed milk, evaporated milk

- **Protein**: Legumes and pulses, some processed meats, poultry and seafood

- **Bread, pasta and cereal products**: Those made from wheat, rye and barley

- **Sugars and sweeteners**: Foods, drinks and snacks containing honey and artificial sweeteners like sorbitol

What foods are low in FODMAPs?

- **Fruit**: Grapes, kiwi fruit, strawberries

- **Vegetables**: Aubergine, carrots, cucumber, peppers, potatoes, tomatoes

- **Dairy and alternatives**: Hard cheeses, lactose-free milk, soya milk made from soya protein

- **Protein**: Eggs, plain cooked meats, poultry and seafood

- **Bread and cereal products**: Wheat-free, barley-free and rye-free breads (although sourdough made with spelt flour is also low-FODMAP)

- **Sugars and sweeteners**: Dark chocolate, table sugar, maple syrup

Where do I start?

If you've ever googled 'IBS and diet' you will know that the FODMAP diet appears high in your search results, with websites listing so-called 'safe' foods, foods to avoid and even recipes.

A word of caution here: although it can be very effective, there is more to the FODMAP diet than simply cutting out offending foods. It is a complex three-stage process that should only be undertaken under the direction of a dietician, who can look at your individual symptoms and dietary needs and support you to follow all three stages of

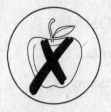 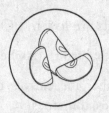 

Restrict high-FODMAP foods and introduce low-FODMAP alternatives

Reintroduce high-FODMAP foods slowly

Personalize your diet for long-term self-management of your symptoms

The three stages of the FODMAP diet

the diet correctly. If you go it alone, you risk missing out on vital nutrients or reintroducing high-FODMAP foods too quickly.

Ask your doctor to refer you to a dietician who specializes in the FODMAP diet. If you want to look for a private practitioner, try searching on the Freelance Dietitians website, which is run in conjunction with the British Dietetic Association (see page 177).

The FODMAP diet is not a one-size-fits-all elimination diet where you cut out all high-FODMAP foods for life. Instead it is a process where, working with a dietician, you identify the FODMAP foods that trigger your symptoms, the ones that have no effect (which you can therefore continue eating) and work out a personalized plan you can follow long-term.

- **Stage 1**: This involves restricting your intake of all high-FODMAP foods for about four to eight weeks, to see if restricting their intake eases your

IBS symptoms. This stage requires organization and discipline in planning what to eat. It is crucial not to deprive yourself of vital vitamins and minerals at this time. You should be looking to substitute high-FODMAP foods with low-FODMAP alternatives – for example, swapping a high-FODMAP onion for chives in recipes.

- **Stage 2**: This stage is all about slowly reintroducing high-FODMAP foods back into your diet. If you find your symptoms have improved in stage one, then you might think it sounds counter-productive to put those very foods that were causing you discomfort and pain back on your plate. However, this stage is crucial in identifying which high-FODMAP foods are causing your issues, and how much you are able to tolerate. A dietician will help guide you through which foods to introduce, when and in what quantities, but you can expect the whole stage to last about eight weeks.

- **Stage 3**: Once the trigger foods have been identified, then you move on to the final stage. The aim here is to work with a dietician who will advise you on how to follow as 'normal' a diet as possible, which is healthy and balanced, but avoids those specific FODMAP foods that trigger your symptoms.

Exercise for IBS

When it comes to exercise, most of us could do with moving about quite a lot more. More than a quarter of the world's adult population (that's about 1.4 billion adults) are insufficiently active.[11]

Exercise has a raft of health benefits: if it came in prescription/tablet form, everyone would ask for it; and yet left to our own devices, we don't seem to embrace it as much as we should. Exercise helps us maintain a healthy weight, is good for our bones and muscles and reduces the risk of cardiovascular disease and cancer. It has significant mental-health benefits as well. But why is exercise so important for people with IBS, and for our gut health in general?

How much – or how little – you move your body affects your GI tract. Physical movement encourages blood flow to the muscles in the GI tract that are involved in peristalsis, helping them to contract and move food along the gut.

Gas is a by-product of digestion, and exercise can help expel gas more quickly. In 2004 eight healthy and exceedingly brave volunteers had a gas mixture pumped into their small intestine, and a catheter placed in their rectums to measure how much gas they passed while pedalling on an exercise bike and while resting. Researchers found that the volunteers released 10 per cent less gas than was pumped into them during a two-hour rest period, yet they released more gas than was pumped in while they were exercising.[12]

Studies involving people with IBS have found that regular exercise can help prevent constipation;[13] there is even some evidence that exercise promotes the growth of gut microbes that help produce short-chain fatty acids. These fatty acids reduce inflammation and can help reduce inflammatory diseases, as well as Type 2 diabetes, obesity and cardiovascular disease.

Many patients that I see are young parents with toddlers who are run off their feet, busy juggling work and childcare. Yet despite this frantic pace, often they are not exercising for themselves. That means at least twenty minutes a day of moderate exercise – to increase the heart rate, become flushed and a little hot, perspire slightly and become slightly out of breath. Just twenty minutes a day would help with their overall energy levels, restore mental resilience and probably help them get a good-quality night's sleep. I always discuss exercise specifically, as it is such an integral part of a healthy life. Avoiding obesity and the associated cancers and ill health are worth the time invested.

And last, but by no means least, are the mental-health benefits of exercise. Exercise also encourages the release of endorphins – 'feel-good' chemicals released by the brain in response to perceived stress or pain. Endorphins act as natural painkillers and affect our mood, making us feel more positive.

How much exercise should I be doing?

According to current guidelines, adults aged nineteen to sixty-four should be aiming for half an hour of moderate-intensity exercise five times a week, plus strength exercises on at least two days a week.[14] Moderate-intensity exercises include brisk walking, hiking, doubles tennis and dancing. Strength exercises include yoga, Pilates, sit-ups and working with resistance bands.

What types of exercise are good for IBS?

Don't get too fixated on what you think you should be doing, but pick something you **want** to do. If you enjoy an activity, you are more likely to stick to it, whether that is a walk each morning before breakfast or a Zoom exercise class with friends. If you are out of practice, start with something gentle, like walking. Other good forms of exercise include:

- Cycling
- Swimming
- Yoga
- Tai chi

Some patients tell me they don't go to the gym any more because of their abdominal symptoms. In this case, even a brisk walk daily or some weight-training exercises will help as you move through treatment plans and symptom management. I am elated any time patients come in and say they are back at the gym or out running again.

Four quick tips to get the most from your workout

1. **Plan your pre- and post-workout meal: Try to avoid any trigger foods before or after exercise.**
2. **Stay hydrated: Stick with water and avoid stimulants like coffee. Likewise, give caffeinated fizzy drinks that could cause gas or loose stools a miss.**
3. **Take any medication that you might need with you.**
4. **Know where the nearest toilet is: If you are exercising outdoors, work out where nearby toilets are when planning your route. The Great British Toilet Map is a website with details of more than 11,000 publicly-accessible toilets across the UK.[15]**

Gut feelings: psychological and holistic therapies for IBS

IBS is a difficult diagnosis and a stressful condition to manage, not only physically but emotionally. It is very common for patients to display classic signs of anxiety and depression.

Often, as we go through their medical history, patients

become emotional and even tearful as they reveal how much their symptoms affect their everyday lives. Some patients even report disciplinary action against them at work, because of absenteeism due to their symptoms. Other people don't realize they are feeling so low until after the treatments work and they think back to how they felt when they first came in. Still others report relationship difficulties, due to their preoccupying gut symptoms and resulting low self-esteem. I have found that highlighting the emotional effects of IBS to my patients can be an eye-opener, because often they don't make the link between their physical symptoms and their mental well-being.

If you have been following medical advice, and prescribed medicines have not helped your symptoms after a year of treatment, you may be offered a referral for what is called 'psychological intervention'. In the UK the National Institute for Health and Care Excellence (NICE) recommends that doctors consider referring patients for this, including hypnotherapy (see page 41) or cognitive behavioural therapy (CBT, see page 44).[16]

One patient of mine, a young man with IBS and abdominal pain, simply didn't respond to the medications we tried. He always had an initial response and felt better, but the symptoms would creep back. After a few months I referred him to a psychology service for talking therapy. After just three sessions he realized he was dealing with his symptoms better, and eventually managed to come off the medication completely and devised an exercise regime that has sustained him for the last three years. Of course he occasionally has some bloating and discomfort, but he is now equipped to manage them.

Some of my patients have also had good results with mindfulness-based therapies (see page 46). I see the journey each patient takes, through the evaluation, treatment trial and subsequent self-management of their symptoms. They become more aware of their own body, its relationship with food and the effect of their mood on symptoms (such as stress-related pain or nausea). Simple mindfulness techniques can enable better control of symptoms, so we may discuss breathing techniques or meditation.

In addition, I often refer patients for hypnotherapy or acupuncture, especially if traditional medical treatments have a limited benefit or are poorly tolerated. Acupuncture is often recommended for people with pain disorders and IBS, and although it doesn't work for everyone, it is a low-risk, safe treatment that can improve the symptoms of pain, anxiety and depression in patients with IBS.[17] A 2020 Chinese randomized controlled trial showed that acupuncture may be more effective than PEG solution (a type of laxative) and an antispasmodic (pinaverium bromide) for the treatment of IBS, with effects lasting up to twelve weeks.[18]

And when it comes to exercise, many patients enjoy relief of their symptoms with regular yoga or Pilates. I believe these benefits all lie within the gut–brain axis and our own ability to down-regulate the way we cope with stress.

Even if you haven't had a formal diagnosis of anxiety or depression, don't dismiss out of hand the offer of a psychological intervention. It is worth accepting a referral or seeking help independently: these are behavioural strategies to help manage your symptoms and condition, and there is good evidence that they can be very beneficial.

It is important to say that not every treatment will suit everyone. If you try something and find it isn't working, go back to your doctor, explain why it isn't working for you and discuss an alternative.

Abdominal breathing technique

Paying attention to your breathing is a simple way to relax your body and help calm a racing mind. Studies show that a deep-breathing technique known as abdominal (or diaphragmatic) breathing can help reduce stress – a key trigger for IBS symptoms.[19]

The diaphragm is a dome-shaped muscle located at the base of the lungs. When we breathe in, the diaphragm contracts and moves the stomach outwards, helping to draw air into the lungs. When we breathe out, the diaphragm relaxes and the stomach flattens once more. Compared to chest-breathing – taking shorter, shallower breaths, such as during vigorous exercise – abdominal breathing is more efficient, allowing more air into the lungs.

Take some time out at the start and end of each day and try this abdominal-breathing exercise. It may feel strange at first, but try not to over-think the action, and persevere: the more you practise, the more natural it will become.

1. Loosen any tight clothing and lie on your back. Keep your knees bent and your feet about 40cm (16 in) apart, with a pillow placed under your knees for support.
2. Gently place your left hand on your chest, and your right hand below your ribcage.
3. Breathe in slowly through the nose, allowing your stomach to rise.
4. Breathe out slowly through pursed lips, allowing your stomach to fall.
5. Repeat for five to ten minutes.

Why sleep matters

Pain, discomfort, needing to go to the toilet, and stress – it is hardly surprising that an estimated 40 per cent of people with IBS have trouble sleeping. IBS has been linked to both poorer-quality sleep and sleep disturbance.

Insomniacs have been found to report more gut problems than good sleepers. Similarly, people with gut complaints report more chronic insomnia than those with a healthy gut. Despite the significant overlap between the two disorders, it is unclear which comes first.

In general I have found that IBS patients complain of taking longer to fall asleep, often because of abdominal discomfort and excessive daytime fatigue. There is, in fact, a documented increase in IBS symptom severity and lower health-related quality-of-life scores linked to poor sleep.

Interestingly, melatonin – a medication used for jet lag and some sleep disorders – has shown some benefit in treating IBS symptoms. Melatonin is produced by the enterochromaffin cells of the digestive tract. There is a higher concentration of melatonin in the gut than in blood or the pineal gland: a pea-shaped gland in the brain whose function isn't fully understood, but which produces and regulates some hormones, including melatonin.

Melatonin has been studied as a potential therapy for IBS, given its role in the regulation of gut motility and possible anti-inflammatory properties. It has been shown to reduce abdominal pain in IBS patients at 3mg daily, but it is not among the therapies for IBS endorsed by a published guideline. Further studies are needed to examine the long-term effect of melatonin, as well as its effect on the central nervous system, sleep and gut motility.

For better sleep quality, try the following suggestions:

- **Avoid heavy meals close to bedtime**: It can take up to eight hours to digest a full meal.

- **Keep your bedtime consistent**: It is really tempting to try to 'catch up' on sleep by having a lie-in at the weekend, but keeping to the same bedtime and wake-up time is crucial in setting a routine.

- **No screens in the bedroom:** Blue light emitted from phones, tablets and televisions can interfere with your circadian rhythm, which is the body's internal clock, making it harder to fall asleep. If you are a light sleeper, you could also think about investing in blackout curtains to keep out the early-morning light.

- **Avoid using alcohol as a sleep aid:** While a couple of glasses of wine may well make you feel more relaxed and drowsy, alcohol affects your sleep cycle, leading to early waking and fatigue the following day.

9. Facing Faecal Facts: What You Need to Know about a Normal Bowel Movement

Poo. Poop. Faeces. Defecation. Answering the call of nature. Whatever you prefer to call it, we all do it. Yet talking about our stool just isn't the done thing in polite company. And so it remains a taboo subject, to be filed away with other so-called embarrassing illnesses and conditions.

Keeping quiet on the subject might be the polite thing to do, but it could be putting your health at risk. We can tell a lot about our general health from our bowel habits, and it is vitally important to know what 'normal' bowel movements feel, look and smell like, so that you are aware of the telltale signs when something isn't right and can seek medical advice.

Coming clean: everything you wanted to know about bowel movements but were too embarrassed to ask

This chapter is all about the things we don't talk about, but should. What colour is a healthy stool – and what indicates a problem? How often should I go to the toilet – and is there a right or wrong way to do so? Here you will find some answers, plus straightforward advice and tips that I hope will de-stigmatize the subject of our stools once and for all.

What exactly is a 'bowel movement'?

Defecation, or having a bowel movement, is the final part of the digestive process and is the act of expelling faeces from our digestive tract via the anus. It is a natural action to expel undigested waste from the foods we eat, as well as metabolic waste products from the body. But while it is natural, having a bowel movement is an extremely complex event, requiring coordination between the gut, brain, nervous system and musculoskeletal system.

And it may surprise you to read that a stool is actually 75 per cent water. The rest is a collection of bacteria and cells from the GI tract, fats, fibre, mucus and bile – the last-named being what gives stool its usual brown colour.

How often should I be having a movement?

This question is one I get asked almost daily, and there is no perfect answer. The range for 'normal' is actually quite broad, but a 2010 study found that 98 per cent of people reported having between three stools per day and three per week.[1]

The frequency of bowel movements can vary due to factors that include age, diet, medication and physical activity. There really is no standard. Probably the most extreme cases I have seen are a patient who hadn't opened her bowels in two weeks, and a man with a particularly severe bout of ulcerative colitis that resulted in twenty trips to the toilet every single day.

What is most important is that you stay in tune with your bowel movements to determine what your individual 'normal' is. So if you suddenly start going a lot more often, or not at all, then it may be time to seek advice.

What colour should my stool be?

This is a really common question that I hear from patients. Stool comes in several shades of brown, green and yellow, all of which are considered normal.

Stool colour is influenced by what we eat, as well as the amount of bile present. As bile pigment travels through the gut, it is chemically altered by enzymes that change the colour from green to brown. However, sometimes stool colour may indicate a serious intestinal condition.

- **Bright-red or burgundy stools**: These colours (as well as black stools, see below) are the most important ones to make us sit up and take notice, because they indicate the presence of blood. Red or burgundy blood is generally from the lower GI tract and reflects a bleeding source within it. This requires prompt medical attention, so contact your family doctor as soon as possible for further investigation.

- **Red stool**: A red stool can be bleeding from a lower-gut source, such as haemorrhoids (piles) or fissures. It can also be due to serious diseases such as colitis or cancer. Foods including red food colouring, beetroot, cranberries, tomato juice or soup, red jelly and drink mixes may cause alarm by producing bright-red stools.

- **Green stool**: This can be due to green leafy vegetables, green food colouring and iron supplements. However, it can also indicate stools moving rapidly through the gut, so that bile doesn't have time to break down.

- **Clay-like or light-coloured stool**: This can be due to some medications, such as Pepto-Bismol. It can also be due to a lack of bile in the stool. It may indicate a bile-duct obstruction around the liver, gall bladder or pancreas.

- **Yellow, greasy or foul-smelling stool**: This is indicative of excess fat in the stool. It may be due to a malabsorption disorder, such as coeliac disease.

- **Black stool**: This can be a sign of bleeding from the stomach, right colon or upper GI tract and is another severe symptom requiring prompt medical attention. You may notice this if you are taking iron supplements, bismuth subsalicylate (kaopectate, Pepto-Bismol) or even black liquorice.

<u>Why does my stool smell so bad?</u>
Stools are not usually associated with a
pleasant odour, but ordinarily it's not
something you tend to sit up and notice. As a
one-off you may notice foul-smelling stools that
are due to something you ate. Again, this is
nothing to concern yourself with.

Our diet affects our stool smell by altering
the gut bacteria. These then produce different
gases, especially sulphur, which has a most
noxious and unpleasant odour. We all know
that an evening indulging in one too many
alcoholic drinks will often result in a smelly,
acidic and mushy stool the following morning,
and this is down to sulphates.

However, sulphur is a necessary element in
our diet, and some foods such as cruciferous
vegetables (broccoli, cabbage, Brussels
sprouts), dairy, eggs and processed meat are
especially effective in increasing our sulphur-
gas expulsion. Certain supplements like
glucosamine and chondroitin are high in
sulphate, which the colonic bacteria convert to
sulphide gases. So the trend is that the more
sulphates that are eaten, the more sulphur is
available for our gut bacteria to make sulphide
gases, which have an offensive odour.

Bad-smelling stools can also indicate a gut
problem. This includes lactose intolerance,
malabsorption of fats from coeliac disease or

pancreatic disease, intestinal infections such as *Clostridium difficile* and inflammatory bowel disease.

The bottom line is: stools can be smelly, but if you notice a persistent smelly-poo problem, it is best to seek advice from your family doctor.

What actually happens during a bowel movement

Defecation is an involuntary process from birth. But from the time we are toilet-trained as toddlers, we learn to control this natural urge to defecate or urinate and do it only when it is socially acceptable to do so. Most of the time we tend not to give our bowel movements much further thought, unless we start to encounter problems in our later years.

During the digestive process the colon transforms liquid stool into the solid faeces you expel when you defecate. Peristalsis (wave-like muscle contractions in the colon) then move the gut contents towards the rectum. As the rectum fills, stretch receptors – clever cells found in muscles that are sensitive to movement – send a signal to the brain of the need to go to the bathroom. But if you are otherwise occupied and defecation is inconvenient – for example, in a meeting or on your morning commute – the rectal wall relaxes and you will temporarily lose the signal.

However, if the time is right to have a bowel movement, you heed the signal and seek out the nearest bathroom. When you sit or squat on the toilet, the abdominal muscles will contract, as well as gradually bearing down. This is the straining feeling you experience when going to the toilet.

The anus has two rings of muscle around it. The inner ring is known as the internal anal sphincter and it remains automatically closed at all times, unless you are having a bowel movement. The outer ring is called the external anal sphincter, which you can voluntarily close if you don't want to defecate – this is the familiar 'squeezing' action you make when holding on until you can make it to the bathroom.

Another muscle involved is the puborectalis, a sling-like muscle that goes from the back of the rectum to the bone at the front of the pelvis. This helps the anus stay closed when you decide that now is not the time for a bowel movement. But when it is, the external anal sphincter and

Are you sitting comfortably? The correct way to sit on the toilet

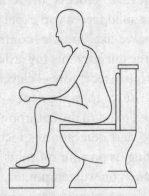

1. Ensure your knees are higher than your hips
2. Lean forward, resting your elbows on your knees
3. Push out your abdomen
4. Straighten your spine

the puborectalis muscle relax, and stool travels from the rectum to the anus and is expelled out of the body.

Is there a right or wrong way to sit on the toilet?

As we now know, there are many factors at play during a bowel movement. But probably the most important action is the relaxation of the puborectalis. Relaxing this muscle opens up what is known as the ano-rectal angle, where the rectum straightens and the pelvis descends to allow for an easier bowel movement.

There has been a lot of discussion in recent years about how our posture affects our bowel movements, and on the need to straighten the ano-rectal angle to allow for a successful bowel movement. In one study researchers compared the use of squat toilets, as used in Asia, the Middle East and South America, to Western toilets, concluding that squat toilets were both more comfortable and more efficient.[2] However, the study only evaluated thirty people, none of whom had bowel problems to begin with.

This new focus on our angle and positioning when we go to the toilet has also led to a burgeoning market in toilet stools, steps and squatty potties to aid defecation. Many people are using toilet stools, which come in a variety of finishes and heights – and you may well have one in your bathroom.

My advice? These devices do create a more favourable angle in the rectal canal, leading to less need to strain. They won't do you any harm, as long as you use them as directed and are otherwise fit and well and have no other issues, such as arthritis or problems with your hips.

Prioritize your bowels: tips for a successful bowel movement every time

- **It's natural, so don't feel embarrassed about it:** The gut–brain axis has highlighted the mind–body connection in relation to bowel movements. There are many people who completely baulk at the idea of using a public toilet, or even facilities at the workplace. Feeling embarrassed is usually the main reason, and a lot of my female patients in particular will admit to this. Having a bowel movement is a natural physical need for all of us. Everybody has to defecate, and there is nothing shameful about this act.

- **Don't rush:** In the same way that you make time to have a shower, brush your teeth or make that first coffee of the day, schedule in toilet time as part of your morning routine. Allow at least ten minutes, ideally after eating breakfast, to utilize the body's natural strongest gut contractions. Silence your phone – and don't be tempted to take it into the toilet with you.

- **Don't put it off:** Repeatedly putting off going to the toilet can lead to constipation, so listen to the 'call to stool'. Try and use the bathroom when you feel the need, instead of holding it in or putting off the bowel movement. Taking advantage of your natural bodily signals and cues will keep your bowels more regular.

- **Relieve that stress**: We know that stress and bowel habits are intricately linked, so try to create a calming private environment in your bathroom.

Utilize stress-relieving activities, such as taking deep breaths, and focus on your body for toilet success.

10. Questions to Ask Your Doctor

Perhaps the most important step in your IBS journey is making that first appointment to see a doctor. If you feel daunted by the prospect, then you aren't alone. Many of my patients will say that they felt nervous before their first appointment.

But remember that an accurate diagnosis will pave the way for the appropriate treatment to enable you to help manage your symptoms. The sooner you get that accurate diagnosis, the sooner that process begins – as well as the relief that will come from discussing your health with a supportive doctor.

It is not uncommon for there to be tears during my first consultation with a patient. The first appointment involves going over intimate details about health, and the impact of symptoms on home, work and social lives. Often there are tears of frustration when recalling previous medical visits, sometimes over a period of years. However, after this first chat is concluded, patients frequently comment that they feel better because they have been listened to and they have a plan, going forward.

A success story

One case in particular stays with me: a woman who had spent five long years seeing her GP and several specialists for her incapacitating diarrhoea.

I could tell, as soon as she set foot in the door, that she was at the end of her tether and our appointment was her last effort at addressing this. After various investigations she turned out to have bile-acid malabsorption and, once on the appropriate treatment, she was back in control of her life. I'll never forget her telling me how she felt like a changed woman, and she was beaming as she left our last consultation.

This chapter is all about preparing you for your initial appointment: practical tips on what you can do beforehand; what you can expect to discuss during your consultation; and the follow-up care you can expect.

If you have been here before and were left dissatisfied with the outcome of your previous appointment, please don't be despondent. You are entitled to a second opinion. Try a different doctor, and use the tips in this chapter to make your next appointment count. A second opinion that results in the right diagnosis could be life-altering.

When is it time to see a doctor?

After reading this book, you are familiar with the symptoms, potential risk factors and treatments that can help manage IBS. No one deserves to put up with the pain and discomfort of IBS.

Ask yourself: are your symptoms affecting your day-to-day life, such as your work, your relationships, your desire to socialize and spend time away from home? Have previous efforts to manage your symptoms been unsuccessful? If the answer is yes, then this is the cue to make an appointment to discuss your health with your doctor.

GP surgery or specialist: what type of doctor should I see?

For the majority of patients, your family doctor will be your first port of call. They should be able to make a diagnosis of IBS, and your initial treatment will usually be overseen by them. If this is not helpful, your GP can refer you to a gastroenterologist. This will happen at the first visit if you display any red-flag symptoms prompting the need for further investigations.

You can also request a referral from your family doctor if you feel that your symptoms are still problematic. The waiting times are very dependent on your local hospital services; or another option is private care. You can also self-refer privately. I always find word-of-mouth recommendations more valuable than searching via websites. You will be surprised to find that many people have experiences with IBS that you may not have been aware of.

A three-stage guide to getting the most out of your appointment

Work through the following stages to give yourself the best chance of making the most of your appointment.

Stage 1: preparation

- **Write it down**: In the run-up to your appointment, get into the habit of making a note of your symptoms – recording the type, frequency and how long you have had them overall. You can then use this to refer to during your appointment, to give your doctor as accurate a picture as possible.

- **Remind yourself of the Rome IV Criteria** in Chapter 1 (see page 18): do your symptoms fall into these criteria? It is also worth reviewing the Bristol Stool Chart (see page 13) to pinpoint the type of stools you typically have. Your doctor should be familiar with this chart: NICE guidelines on diagnosing and managing IBS recommend that health professionals use it to help to establish bowel habit.[1]

- **Don't forget to record the impact of your symptoms on your quality of life**: Has a need to be near a toilet meant that long car journeys are fraught with anxiety? Or does your abdominal pain drive you to distraction during your working day? Tell your doctor about it, so they can build up a full picture of how your symptoms affect you.

- **Mention your diet and medication**: Have you tried an exclusion diet? If so, note down what you typically eat in a day, what you have excluded and whether it has had any impact. And bring with you a list of current medication, including any over-the-counter or herbal medicines.

- **Have a lot to discuss? Request a double appointment**: A 2017 study found that the UK has the shortest GP consultations in Europe, with British patients spending just over nine minutes with their GP.[2] If your medical history is long, your symptoms are extensive or you simply feel you need extra time, it could be worth asking for a double appointment.

Stage 2: during the appointment

- **Need some support? Ask to bring a friend**: If you are feeling apprehensive, having a trusted friend or partner can help. Make sure it is **you** taking the lead in describing your symptoms, but discuss beforehand with your friend the main points you want to talk about in your consultation, so that they can prompt you if you forget to mention something important.

- **What you should expect to discuss**: A full and frank conversation of your symptoms is crucial: what they are, when they occur and how long you have been experiencing them, plus their effect on your quality of life. You should also be asked about your family medical history, your current diet and any medication you take.

  Please don't feel embarrassed to talk about your bowel habits. It is thought that about 20 per cent of people experiencing faecal incontinence disclose their incontinence only if asked.[3] Doctors are highly trained and, believe me, we will have heard it all before. We need a full picture in order to make the right diagnosis and treatment recommendations.

- **Will I need a physical examination?**: Your doctor will want to examine you, including an abdominal check for any tenderness or distension. If you have had rectal bleeding, you may need a rectal examination, which can be slightly daunting, but it is a simple and quick exam.

- **What tests might I have?**: You may have the following blood tests:

  ○ **Full blood count (FBC)** is a very common screening test used to diagnose and monitor a

155

number of conditions.[4] The FBC looks at the types and numbers of cells in your blood, including red blood cells, white blood cells and platelets. An elevated number of white blood cells is called leucocytosis, which can be down to bacterial infections or inflammation. A low white-blood-cell count is called leucopenia and can be due to causes including viral infections.

○ **Erythrocyte sedimentation rate (ESR)** can diagnose conditions associated with inflammation, such as Crohn's disease. It measures how long it takes for red blood cells to fall to the bottom of a test tube. The quicker they fall, the more likely it is there are high levels of inflammation.

○ **C-reactive protein (CRP)** is a blood test used to help diagnose conditions that cause inflammation. CRP is a protein produced by the liver: a high concentration indicates inflammation.

○ **Total immunoglobulin A (IgA) and IgA Tissue transglutaminase antibody (tTG) blood tests** look for antibodies present in the bloodstream of people with coeliac disease.[5] They are accurate only if you have been ingesting gluten in the preceding months, so do make your doctor aware if you are excluding this.

○ **Other blood tests** may be requested, depending on your specific symptoms – for instance, tests to check thyroid function. You may also be asked to bring in a stool sample to check for infection or hidden blood.

Stage 3: what next?

Once you have been diagnosed with IBS, your doctor should talk to you about potential treatments. This should be guided by the nature and severity of your symptoms. The conversation should also cover the importance of self-help in effectively managing your IBS, including information on your general lifestyle, physical activity and diet.

Before the appointment ends, establish what your treatment plan is and when you should book in for a follow-up appointment. IBS is rarely dealt with in just a few visits. Instead it may take several months to fully manage your symptoms. The constant review and tweaking of treatments will provide optimal success in the end.

If you are unsure about anything, don't be afraid to ask questions. As a professional, I would much rather that patients are clear on the course of action before they leave the room. It is important to voice any concerns about your symptoms, because everyone is different. For some people it might be a desire not to feel uncomfortable and bloated for their upcoming wedding; for others, it might be the embarrassment of needing the toilet frequently whilst at work; and for yet others, the loud, irrepressible burps after eating that affect their social life.

Asking for a second opinion – and what to do if your treatment isn't working

If you are not satisfied with the outcome of the appointment, speak up. It is important that a consultation is a two-way thing and you are entitled to ask for a second opinion, whether that is from another doctor at the same surgery or requesting a specialist referral.

Likewise, if you feel your treatment plan isn't helping, or if your symptoms worsen – even with medication – go back, build a rapport with your doctor and push for a specialist referral. You don't have to go with the person your GP recommends, when you ask for a referral. You can do your own research, and again word-of-mouth and personal recommendation are always good options.

Ten key questions to ask your doctor

1. **Do I need a referral to a gastroenterologist?**
2. **Are there any over-the-counter treatments that can help my symptoms?**
3. **What about my diet – should I be doing anything different?**
4. **What are the benefits and risks of the treatments you have prescribed?**
5. **Are there any side-effects that I should be aware of?**
6. **How soon can I expect my symptoms to improve?**

7. Do I need to come back and see you? If so, when?
8. Who do I contact if my symptoms change or get worse?
9. What red-flag symptoms of other conditions should I be looking out for?
10. Is there a support group or any other source of help?

Conclusion

We are at the beginning of the road towards a bright future for those suffering from IBS. We can now embrace the explosion of gut-microbiome research and apply it effectively, as we move forward in our understanding and acceptance of IBS. No longer deemed 'functional' and unworthy of medical attention, IBS has finally entered its spotlight moment of recognition and, more importantly, acknowledgement.

I wanted to write this book for the many frustrated, emotional, ignored, fobbed-off people I have seen who eventually became empowered, smiling, positive, relieved and confident wives, husbands, daughters, sons and family members again. I am hopeful for each and every one of my patients, and for each person who reads this book and realizes there are always options available.

I truly believe it speaks volumes that in December 2020 we saw the first-ever American College of Gastroenterology clinical guidelines for the management of IBS. This was closely followed in April 2021 by the British Society of Gastroenterology guidelines on the management of IBS, which had not been updated since 2007. Even more positively, there is a recommendation to review these guidelines every four years now, rather than the fourteen years that have passed. I am extremely excited to see what future treatment options will be available to us.

The guidelines did make me reminisce on my medical-school days, when we were initially taught to take a detailed history and to examine our patients. It seems that many doctors have forgotten this rudimentary skill, as the 2021 guidelines stress these simple facts yet again. The key to any success, in medical terms, is the doctor–patient relationship, and it is not one that ends at the first consultation. This is a journey that you should take with a doctor who wants to understand you, your condition and your concerns, and who provides continuity in your care.

Yes, IBS is a positive diagnosis. Yes, IBS doesn't kill us. Yes, people with IBS can get other diseases and need to listen to their own bodies, and be listened to very closely when seeking medical advice.

We can look forward to tailored individual care to address our diet, exercise, mental health and microbiome. Eventually our gut will provide precious insights into our overall state of health. I hope this book will empower you to move forward and take charge of your IBS and of your wider health.

I'd like to leave you with five quotes from Hippocrates, the 'father of medicine', whom I believe to be a gastroenterologist at heart. Perhaps they will give you food for thought – something to chew over mentally – but also the grounding principle to listen to your gut feelings:

1. All disease starts in the gut.

2. Just as food causes chronic disease, it can be the most powerful cure.

3. It's far more important to know what sort of person the disease has than what sort of disease the person has.

4. The patient must combat the disease along with the physician.

5. Let food be thy medicine, and medicine be thy food.

Notes

1. Inside Our Digestive System, and Understanding IBS

1 C. Canavan et al. (2014), 'Review article: The economic impact of the irritable bowel syndrome', *Alimentary Pharmacology and Therapeutics*, 40 (9), pp.1023–34, doi.org/10.1111/apt.12938

2 S. L. Shah et al. (2021), 'Patients With Irritable Bowel Syndrome Are Willing to Take Substantial Medication Risks for Symptom Relief', *Clinical Gastroenterology and Hepatology: The Official Clinical Practice Journal of the American Gastroenterological Association*, 19 (1), pp.80–86, doi.org/10.1016/j.cgh.2020.04.003

3 Canavan et al. (2014), 'Review article: The economic impact of the irritable bowel syndrome'

2. IBS Risk Factors

1 T. Iacon, D. F. Țățulescu, M. S. Lupse, D. L. Dumitrașcu (2020), 'Post-infectious irritable bowel syndrome after a laboratory-proven enteritis', *Experimental and Therapeutic Medicine*, 20 (4), pp.3517–22, doi.org/10.3892/etm.2020.9018

3. The Gut–Brain Axis Explained

1 K. Bradford et al. (2012), 'Association between early adverse life events and irritable bowel syndrome', *Clinical Gastroenterology and Hepatology*, 10 (4), pp.385–90

2 C. Flik et al. (2018), 'Efficacy of individual and group hypnotherapy in irritable bowel syndrome (IMAGINE): A multicentre randomised controlled trial', *The Lancet Gastroenterology and Hepatology*, 4 (1), pp.20–31, doi.org/10.1016/S2468-1253(18)30310-8

3 National Council for Hypnotherapy, 'Hypnotherapy for IBS', www.hypnotherapists.org.uk/hypnotherapy/hypnotherapy-for-ibs/

4 S. Ballou and L. Keefer (2017), 'Psychological Interventions for Irritable Bowel Syndrome and Inflammatory Bowel Diseases', *Clinical and Translational Gastroenterology*, 8 (1), e214

5 J. M. Lackner, J. Jaccard, S. S. Krasner et al. (2008), 'Self-administered cognitive behavior therapy for moderate to severe irritable bowel syndrome: Clinical efficacy, tolerability, feasibility', *Clinical Gastroenterology and Hepatology*, 6 (8), pp.899–906

6 Bold Health's Zemedy, www.zemedy.com

7 Mindset Nerva, www.mindsethealth.com/nerva

8 B. D. Naliboff et al. (2020), 'Mindfulness-based stress reduction improves irritable bowel syndrome (IBS) symptoms via specific aspects of mindfulness', *Neurogastroenterology and Motility: The official journal of the European Gastrointestinal Motility Society*, 32 (9), e13828, doi.org/10.1111/nmo.13828

4. Alarm Symptoms: When Are My Sympstoms Not Down to IBS?

1 L. Watson et al. (2015), 'Management of bile acid malabsorption using low-fat dietary interventions: A useful strategy applicable to some patients with diarrhoea-predominant irritable bowel syndrome?', *Clinical Medicine*, 15 (6), pp.536–40

2 World Cancer Research Fund, 'Ovarian Cancer Statistics', www.wcrf.org/dietandcancer/ovarian-cancer-statistics/

3 World Cancer Research Fund, 'Colorectal Cancer Statistics', www.wcrf.org/dietandcancer/colorectal-cancer-statistics/

5. Associated Conditions

1 W. E. Whitehead, O. S. Palsson, R. R. Levy et al. (2007), 'Comorbidity in irritable bowel syndrome', *American Journal of Gastroenterology*, 102, pp.2767–76

2 A. Mulak and L. Paradowski (2005), '*Migrena a zespół jelita nadwrazliwego*' ['Migraine and irritable bowel syndrome'], *Neurologia i Neurochirurgia Polska*, 39 (4), pp.S55–60

3 L. A. Houghton et al. (2002), 'The menstrual cycle affects rectal sensitivity in patients with irritable bowel syndrome but not healthy volunteers', *Gut*, 50 (4), pp.471–4

6. The Gut Microbiome Explained

1 Heathrow.com, 'Traffic and passenger statistics', www.heathrow.com/company/about-heathrow/performance/airport-operations/traffic-statistics

2 M. Levy et al. (2017), 'Dysbiosis and the immune system', *Nature Reviews: Immunology*, 17 (4), pp.219–32

3 W. L. Wang, S. Y. Xu, Z. G. Ren et al. (2015), 'Application of metagenomics in the human gut microbiome', *World Journal of Gastroenterology*, 21 (3), pp.803–14

4 R. Ortigão et al. (2020), 'Gastrointestinal Microbiome – What We Need to Know in Clinical Practice', *GE Portuguese Journal of Gastroenterology*, 27 (5), pp.336–51, doi.org/10.1159/000505036

5 G. Sisson et al. (2014), 'Randomised clinical trial: A liquid multi-strain probiotic vs. placebo in the irritable bowel syndrome – a 12 week double-blind study', *Alimentary Pharmacology & Therapeutics*, 40 (1), pp.51–62

7. Symptom-Based Medication Treatment

1 G. Istre et al. (1982), 'An outbreak of amebiasis spread by colonic irrigation at a chiropractic clinic', *The New England Journal of Medicine*, 307 (6), pp.339–42

2 E. D. Shah, H. M. Kim and P. Schoenfeld (2018), 'Efficacy and Tolerability of Guanylate Cyclase-C Agonists for Irritable Bowel Syndrome with Constipation and Chronic Idiopathic Constipation: A Systematic Review and Meta-Analysis', *American Journal of Gastroenterology*, 113 (3), pp.329–38

3 C. M. Prather et al. (2000), 'Tegaserod accelerates orocecal transit in patients with constipation-predominant irritable bowel syndrome', *Gastroenterology*, 118 (3), pp.463–8, doi.org/10.1016/s0016-5085(00)70251-4

4 E. P. Bouras, M. Camilleri, D. D. Burton et al. (1999), 'Selective stimulation of colonic transit by the benzofuran 5HT4 agonist, prucalopride, in healthy humans', *Gut*, 44, pp.682–6

5 T. S. Odunsi-Shiyanbade et al. (2010), 'Effects of chenodeoxycholate and a bile acid sequestrant, colesevelam, on intestinal transit and bowel function', *Clinical Gastroenterology and Hepatology*, 8 (2), pp.159–65

6 V. Andresen et al. (2008), 'Effects of 5-hydroxytryptamine (serotonin) type 3 antagonists on symptom relief and constipation in nonconstipated irritable bowel syndrome: A systematic review and meta-analysis of randomized controlled trials', *Clinical Gastroenterology and Hepatology*, 6 (5), pp.545–55

7 M. Camilleri, A. C. Ford (2017), 'Pharmacotherapy for Irritable Bowel Syndrome', *Journal of Clinical Medicine*, 6 (11), doi.org/10.3390/jcm6110101

8 A. C. Ford, N. J. Talley, P. S. Schoenfeld et al. (2009), 'Efficacy of antidepressants and psychological therapies in irritable bowel syndrome: Systematic review and meta-analysis', *Gut*, 58 (3), pp.367–78

9 R. A. Moore et al. (2015), 'Amitriptyline for neuropathic pain in adults', *Cochrane Database of Systematic Reviews*, doi.org/10.1002/14651858.CD008242.pub3

10 G. Tabas, M. Beaves, J. Wang et al. (2004), 'Paroxetine to treat irritable bowel syndrome not responding to high-fiber diet: A double-blind, placebo-controlled trial', *American Journal of Gastroenterology*, 99, p.914.

11 M. Pimentel et al. (2011), 'Rifaximin therapy for patients with irritable bowel syndrome without constipation', *The*

New England Journal of Medicine, 364 (1), pp.22–32, doi.org/
10.1056/NEJMoa1004409

12 S. B. Menees et al. (2021), 'The efficacy and safety of rifaximin for the irritable bowel syndrome: A systematic review
and meta-analysis', *American Journal of Gastroenterology*, 107
(1), pp.28–35; quiz p.36

8. Dietary and Psychological Treatments

1 M. Simrén et al. (2001), 'Food-related gastrointestinal symptoms in the irritable bowel syndrome', *Digestion*, 63 (2), pp.
108–15

2 Ibid.

3 S. S. Khayyatzadeh et al. (2018), 'Dietary behaviors in relation
to prevalence of irritable bowel syndrome in adolescent girls',
Journal of Gastroenterology and Hepatology, 33 (2), pp.404–10

4 Gloucestershire Hospitals NHS Foundation Trust (2020),
'Fluid and caffeine intake for bladder and bowel health',
www.gloshospitals.nhs.uk/media/documents/Fluid_and_
caffeine_intake_for_bladder_and_bowel_health_GHPI
0533_02_20.pdf

5 C. J. Derry, S. Derry, R. A. Moore (2014), 'Caffeine as an analgesic adjuvant for acute pain in adults', *Cochrane Database
of Systematic Reviews*, doi.org/10.1002/14651858.CD009281.
pub2

6 NHS.uk (2018), 'Alcohol Units', www.nhs.uk/live-well/
alcohol-support/calculating-alcohol-units/#:~:text=
men%20and%20women%20are%20advised,as%2014%20
units%20a%20week

7 D. H. Vasant, P. A. Paine, C. J. Black et al. (2021), 'British Society of Gastroenterology guidelines on the management of irritable bowel syndrome', *Gut*, doi.org/10.1136/gutjnl-2021-324598

8 L. Schnabel et al. (2018), 'Association Between Ultra-Processed Food Consumption and Functional Gastrointestinal Disorders: Results from the French Nutri Net-Santé Cohort', *American Journal of Gastroenterology*, 113 (8), pp.1217–28

9 N. Alammar et al. (2019), 'The impact of peppermint oil on the irritable bowel syndrome: A meta-analysis of the pooled clinical data', *BMC Complementary and Alternative Medicine*, 19 (1), doi.org/10.1186/s12906-018-2409-0

10 R. Khanna, J. K. MacDonald and B. G. Levesque (2014), 'Peppermint oil for the treatment of irritable bowel syndrome: A systematic review and meta-analysis', *Journal of Clinical Gastroenterology*, 48 (6), pp.505–12

11 World Health Organization (2020), 'Physical activity', www.who.int/news-room/fact-sheets/detail/physical-activity#:~:text=Adults%20aged%2018%%E2%80%9364%20years&text=may%20increase%20moderate%2Dintensity%20aerobic,week%20for%20additional%20health%20benefits

12 R. Dainese et al. (2004), 'Effects of physical activity on intestinal gas transit and evacuation in healthy subjects', *American Journal of Medicine*, 116 (8), pp.536–9, doi.org/10.1016/j.amjmed.2003.12.018

13 A. J. Daley et al. (2008), 'The effects of exercise upon symptoms and quality of life in patients diagnosed with irritable

bowel syndrome: A randomised controlled trial', *International Journal of Sports Medicine*, 29 (9), pp.778–82

14 NHS.uk, 'Exercise', www.nhs.uk/live-well/exercise/

15 Great British Toilet Map, www.toiletmap.org.uk

16 NICE (2008), 'Irritable bowel syndrome in adults: Diagnosis and management', www.nice.org.uk/guidance/cg61

17 Rome Foundation, 'Acupuncture Treatment for the Disorders of Gut–Brain Interaction (DGBI): A Report from China', www.theromefoundation.org/acupuncture-treatment-for-dgbi/

18 L. Pei, H. Geng, J. Guo et al. (2020), 'Effect of Acupuncture in Patients With Irritable Bowel Syndrome: A Randomized Controlled Trial', *Mayo Clinic Proceedings*, 95 (8), pp.1671–83

19 X. Ma et al. (2017), 'The Effect of Diaphragmatic Breathing on Attention, Negative Affect and Stress in Healthy Adults', *Frontiers in Psychology*, 8, doi.org/10.3389/fpsyg.2017.00874

9. Facing Faecal Facts:
What You Need to Know about a Normal Bowel Movement

1 S. A. Walter et al. (2010), 'Assessment of normal bowel habits in the general adult population: The Popcol study', *Scandinavian Journal of Gastroenterology*, 45 (5), pp.556–66, doi.org/10.3109/00365520903551332

2 D. Sikirov (2003), 'Comparison of straining during defecation in three positions: Results and implications for human health', *Digestive Diseases and Sciences*, 48 (7), pp.1201–5, doi.org/10.1023/a:1024180319005

10. Questions to Ask Your Doctor

1 National Institute for Health and Care Excellence (2017), 'Irritable bowel syndrome in adults: Diagnosis and management', www.nice.org.uk/guidance/cg61

2 G. Irving, A. L. Neves, H. Dambha-Miller et al. (2017), 'International variations in primary care physician consultation time: A systematic review of 67 countries', *British Medical Journal Open*, 7 (10), doi.org/10.1136/bmjopen-2017-017902

3 NICE (2017), 'Irritable bowel syndrome in adults: Diagnosis and management', www.nice.org.uk/guidance/cg61

4 Association for Clinical Biochemistry and Laboratory Medicine (2020), 'Full Blood Count (FBC)', labtestsonline.org.uk/tests/full-blood-count-fbc

5 NHS.uk (2018), 'Examples: Blood tests', www.nhs.uk/conditions/blood-tests/types/

Further Reading and Resources

General information on IBS and other functional gut disorders

Asian Pacific Association of Gastroenterology (APAGE), www.apage.org, a professional organization

Badgut.org, www.badgut.org, information on gastrointestinal and liver conditions from the Canadian Society of Intestinal Research

Canadian Digestive Health Foundation, www.cdhf.ca, information and up-to-date research on IBS and other digestive conditions for people living in Canada

Gastroenterological Society of Australia, www.GESA.org.au, a professional organization that also has patient information resources

Guts UK, www.gutscharity.org.uk, a UK charity for digestive disorders

IBS Network, www.theibsnetwork.org, a UK IBS charity

Indian Society of Gastroenterology, www.isg.org.in, a professional organization

International Foundation for Functional Gastrointestinal Disorders, www.aboutibs.org, a US-based charity

Pakistan Society of Gastroenterology and GI Endoscopy, www.psgpak.org, professional organization

Rome Foundation, www.theromefoundation.org, an organization that aims to improve the lives of people with functional GI disorders

South African Gastroenterology Society, www.sages.co.za, a professional organization that includes patient information

United European Gastroenterology, www.ueg.eu, a professional non-profit organization of European medical specialists and national societies, focusing on digestive health

IBS Guidelines

American College of Gastroenterology, *ACG Clinical Guideline: Management of Irritable Bowel Syndrome*, journals.lww.com/ajg/Fulltext/2021/01000/ACG_Clinical_Guideline__Management_of_Irritable.11.aspx

British Society of Gastroenterology, *Guidelines on the Management of Irritable Bowel Syndrome*, www.bsg.org.uk/clinical-resource/british-society-of-gastroenterology-guidelines-on-the-management-of-irritable-bowel-syndrome/

National Institute for Health and Care Excellence (NICE), *Irritable bowel syndrome in adults: Diagnosis and management* (last updated 2017), www.nice.org.uk/guidance/cg61

IBS treatment and lifestyle

British Association for Behavioural and Cognitive Psychotherapies, www.cbtregisteruk.com, a list of accredited CBT therapists

British Association of Mindfulness-Based Approaches, www.
bamba.org.uk, a list of qualified mindfulness teachers

British Dietetic Association Freelance Dietitians Group, www.
freelancedietitians.org, directory of registered dieticians

King's College London, www.kcl.ac.uk/lsm/Schools/life-course-
sciences/departments/nutritional-sciences/projects/
fodmaps, the low-FODMAP diet adapted by researchers
for the UK

Monash Low FODMAP Diet, www.monashfodmap.com,
website of Monash University, Australia, founders of the
low-FODMAP diet

National Council for Hypnotherapy (NCH), www.hypnother-
apists.org.uk/therapist-finder, a list of NCH-registered
hypnotherapists

Helpful patient information websites

Brazilian Federation of Gastroenterology, www.campanhas.
fbg.org.br/saude-digestiva, a patient information website

Mayo Clinic, www.mayoclinic.org/patient-care-and-health-
information, information on conditions and treatments
from the US-based, non-profit health organization

MedlinePlus, www.medlineplus.gov, health-information websites from the US National Library of Medicine

Patient, www.patient.info, a symptom checker and health information reviewed by UK health professionals

Acknowledgements

I am truly excited about removing the word 'just' from before the diagnosis of IBS and, hopefully, giving millions of sufferers true validation. I wish to thank all of the patients whom I have encountered over the years, not only in providing me with challenging experiences, but also in learning through exceptional journeys together.

I would very much like to thank Lydia Yadi, Susannah Bennett and Kat Keogh at Penguin Random House for this opportunity to highlight irritable bowel syndrome. Their enthusiasm and expert guidance in writing this book have allowed me to express my own experience in this medical field over the last decade – and much is changing for the positive.

This project would not have been possible without the inspiration, teaching and mentoring I have enjoyed through medical school at Guy's Hospital in London, the beginning of my learning. I would like to thank my medical residency teams at Boston City Hospital for fostering my interest in gastroenterology. I am most grateful to Columbia Medical Center Gastroenterology Division for providing an exceptional fellowship training, which is still second to none. My peers, colleagues and attendings at Columbia shaped my subsequent path in this broad and varied speciality. Back then, coeliac disease was deemed a rarity! I am indebted to my previous gastro team at the Royal London Hospital, whose foresight enabled me to become the first Community Consultant Gastroenterologist in the UK, allowing focus on improved, efficient, seamless, joined-up outpatient care for IBS (and, hopefully, other gut conditions) as well as endoscopy. I am optimistic that this will change the entire patient experience in the future. I would also like to acknowledge recent colleagues who inadvertently made me realize that a well-rounded experience is indeed invaluable.

I must extend my special thanks to my beloved mum and dad, Dr Umapada and Manjusree Das, for their unfaltering support, patience and loving encouragement throughout my medical career. Without them, I doubt I would be enjoying this wonderful writing opportunity. I only wish I could share this with them now. My loving thanks also extend to my two fabulous daughters, Corinna and Katarina, who have tirelessly and (almost) non-complainingly listened to my ravings about the beauty of the small intestine, picturesque polyps and the newly discovered gut microbiome and its pluripotential. They have read and reread my drafts and helped to shape the various chapters. I trust they have gained from this experience, too.

Finally, I would like to say thank you to my fabulous friends Dr Esther Valdez and Georginna Summers for listening, supporting and inspiring me to keep up my passion to serve my patients holistically. My gratitude goes also to the many female consultant friends and colleagues who quietly understand and support the extra perseverance needed in our daily lives.

I have thoroughly enjoyed writing this book and hope that many will find it a rewarding read.

PREPARING FOR THE PERIMENOPAUSE AND MENOPAUSE

DR LOUISE NEWSON

The *Sunday Times* Number One Bestseller.

Part of the Penguin Life Experts series.

Dr Louise Newson is the UK's leading menopause specialist, and she's determined to help women thrive during the menopause.

Despite being something that almost every woman will experience at some point in their lives, menopause is frequently misdiagnosed and misinformation and stigma are commonplace. Dr Newson demystifies the menopause and explains why every woman should be perimenopause-aware, regardless of their age.

Using new research, expert advice and empowering patient stories from a diverse range of women who have struggled to secure adequate treatment and correct diagnosis, Dr Newson equips readers with expert advice and practical tips. She empowers women to confidently take charge of their health and their changing bodies.

It's never too early to learn about the perimenopause or menopause and this compact guide will provide you with everything you need to know.

UNDERSTANDING ALLERGY
DR SOPHIE FAROOQUE

Part of the Penguin Life Experts series.

One in three of us experience allergies at some point in our lives and we are more allergic than ever before, so why are allergies still so misunderstood?

Dr Sophie Farooque, a leading expert and consultant in allergy, will provide allergy sufferers and their families with the knowledge they need to help them navigate this minefield. *Understanding Allergy* offers practical advice to reduce unnecessary suffering and debunk common allergy myths.

MANAGING YOUR MIGRAINE
DR KATY MUNRO

Part of the Penguin Life Experts series.

Despite being one of the most common and debilitating conditions in the world, migraine is still widely misunderstood, stigmatized and misdiagnosed. Migraine is much more than 'just a headache', so why do we still know so little about this genetic neurological brain disorder and its causes? Headache specialist and GP Dr Katy Munro has the answers you're looking for.

Managing Your Migraine is the practical go-to guide for understanding migraine, equipping readers with practical, expert advice.

If you're a person with migraine, or know someone struggling, this book will provide helpful strategies for alleviating and managing your symptoms. Drawing on her medical expertise, her own personal experience with migraine and the stories of her patients, Dr Munro will empower you to get to know your own migraine and build an effective treatment plan that will help you to live your life to the full.